The Diabetes Manifesto

The Diabetes Manifesto

Take Charge of Your Life

Lynn Crowe

Julie Stachowiak, PhD

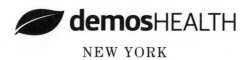

NEW YORK

Acquisitions Editor: Noreen Henson
Cover Design: Carlos Maldonado
Compositor: Absolute Service, Inc.
Printer: Hamiton Printing Company

Visit our website at www.demoshealth.com

Medical information provided by Demos Health, in the absence of a visit with a health care professional, must be considered as an educational service only. This book is not designed to replace a physician's independent judgment about the appropriateness or risks of a procedure or therapy for a given patient. Our purpose is to provide you with information that will help you make your own health care decisions.

The information and opinions provided here are believed to be accurate and sound, based on the best judgment available to the authors, editors, and publisher, but readers who fail to consult appropriate health authorities assume the risk of any injuries. The publisher is not responsible for errors or omissions. The editors and publisher welcome any reader to report to the publisher any discrepancies or inaccuracies noticed.

Library of Congress Cataloging-in-Publication Data

Crowe, Lynn.
  The diabetes manifesto : take charge of your life / Lynn Crowe, Julie Stachowiak.
    p. cm.
  Includes bibliographical references and index.
  ISBN 978-1-932603-94-1
  1. Diabetes—Popular works. 2. Diabetes—Psychological aspects. I. Stachowiak, Julie. II. Title.
  RC660.4.C76 2011
  616.4'62—dc22

                          2010038543

Made in the United States of America
10 11 12 13   5 4 3 2 1

Contents

Introduction: The Manifesto

This is a book about dignity.

More specifically, this book is about living with dignity while simultaneously dealing with diabetes. Like many chronic diseases, diabetes can eradicate our sense of control and our self-esteem if we are not actively fighting to keep ourselves whole every moment. However, diabetes comes with some extra challenges to maintaining our confidence in our choices and ourselves.

Diabetes comes with a lion's share of blame and guilt. The blame comes from others (including doctors) because they often believe that we did this to ourselves (in the case of type 2 diabetes), that any complication that comes along indicates that we were not vigilant in following treatment plans, any blood glucose reading that is a little high is proof that we are not trying hard enough or that we gave into temptation because of a lack of willpower. The guilt comes because maybe we believe them, if even just a little bit.

This, my friends, is bullshit.

It is my goal to bring you information and ideas that give you a healthy perspective on living with diabetes, balancing hope with realism.

To clarify, we are all still accountable for our actions and for the impact of our actions on our diabetes. Yes, we need to work like hell to stay healthy (many of us more than others) and, no, it is not "fair" (whatever that means) that we have this burden and others don't. However, one of my goals in this book is to put things in perspective. We need to get away from the black and white equation that tight glucose control equals a life free from diabetes-related complications. For many of us, complications enter our lives, despite our efforts. Because the threat of complications has been used as "motivation" to keep us compliant to treatment, not only do we feel shame at our "failure" to keep complications away, but also we are terrified of them. Another important part of my message is that complications are not a death sentence. They can be managed, just like we manage our diabetes.

So, while I am telling you that only part of diabetes is under anyone's control, I also want to emphasize that we *do* need to constantly be taking action to try to keep our blood glucose within our target range—striving for *accountability* for our decisions and actions *without shame* around any diabetes-related problems. I, personally, have decided that my best shot is to do my best to attain ideal glucose levels without totally sacrificing my life and becoming a walking disease, unable to think or talk about anything else. Living with diabetes is about vigilance and balance. Even though I cannot realistically maintain ideal blood glucose levels, I work toward that goal, knowing that perfectionism in diabetes is a losing battle. It is a challenge every day.

Which brings us back to dignity—dignity is about quality of life, which can be defined as "the degree to which a person enjoys the important possibilities of his or her life."[1] To that end, *The Diabetes Manifesto* will take you through different aspects of life with diabetes, in search of ways to increase the possibilities of your life. This includes optimizing medical care and managing complications, but also extends to relationships, emotions, activism, and much more. In each of these areas, *The Diabetes Manifesto* will help you to figure out what you need, identify opportunities, understand the challenges, and get your needs met.

Take Charge

Decide to be a person living with diabetes, armed with knowledge and confidence, who is prepared to take action.

Each Person's Diabetes is Personal

We know that there are two primary types of diabetes, and some other, less common, types. To complicate matters, even within the different types, we all have different disease paths. Even among people sharing

---

[1] Definition of quality of life from the Quality of Life Research Unit of the University of Toronto.

a complication, the spectrum is huge—what is an annoyance to one person can strike another person much harder and become disabling.

Despite these differences, there are things that make us similar as people living with diabetes. We can't say for sure what the future holds. We really don't know what our next complication might be or when it will show up. We don't know which medications or procedures will help us feel better until we try them.

We do know that we didn't do anything to cause the diabetes, even though there are some contributing factors to type 2 diabetes. And, sadly, we know that, for the moment, there is no cure for diabetes. Most of all, we know that we would really rather not have diabetes.

For People With Diabetes, by a Person With Diabetes

As a person who is living with type 1 diabetes, admittedly some days more successfully than others, I want to share with you what has worked to keep me going. To keep me from losing my confidence, and to preserve those parts of myself that I take pride in. I have tried to capture the essence of my strategies and feelings in the pages of this book.

We now know a great deal more about other aspects of diabetes and the tools we have to manage diabetes are light-years from where they were when I was diagnosed as a child. I am fortunate to have these tools at my disposal today, but often wonder where I would be in terms of complications if they had been in my arsenal since day one. However, I know that there is much more for the scientists to learn about treating diabetes and preventing complications—in terms of a "cure" or a way to manage this disease free of complications, we are not there yet.

I work in the pharmaceutical industry, namely helping people with type 2 diabetes transition to insulin. I run across a great deal of information written by "experts" who discuss what diabetes patients, sufferers, or victims *should* do, with promises that if the instructions are followed, they will *never* have to worry about any of those yucky complications.

There is a great deal of misguided blame around diabetes. Too many people look at the disease and its complications through a "cause-and-effect" filter that is inaccurate. This results in people becoming "failures" in the business of life. That is simply unacceptable to me, as it hands power over to this disease that we are trying to fight.

> **The Real World**
>
> Okay, diabetes sucks. It truly does. Let's just get that out there.

My Manifesto

I was diagnosed with type 1 diabetes when I was 12 years old. Even at that young age, I was already familiar with diabetes. About a year and a half earlier, my older brother was admitted to the hospital for fatigue and other strange symptoms and emerged as a person with diabetes.

For a young girl, the implications of my brother's diagnosis were more interesting than alarming to me. He monitored his "sugar" by urinating into little beakers. It was all very scientific and interesting, in my opinion. My parents responded to his diagnosis by making sure there was always an abundance of fresh fruits in the house—in the early 1970s, we knew nothing of appropriate carbohydrate to insulin ratios.

My first symptoms were constant cravings for fluids and seemingly nonstop urination; more precisely, "peeing my brains out." Nobody seemed too alarmed. After all, my parents had been reassured repeatedly by the doctor that there was no chance that any of their other children would be diagnosed with diabetes. Much to my naive delight, I proved them all wrong by using one of my brother's testing beakers to demonstrate my scientific prowess and show that my sugar was indeed off the charts. This preteen glee quickly turned into a frantic trip to the hospital, where I was admitted with full-blown diabetic ketoacidosis (a life-threatening condition) and blood glucose levels around 1100 mg/dL.

Thirty-seven years have passed. I am a person living with diabetes.

These years have not been smooth. I have learned not to simply fear this illness, but to respect what it can do to me and what I (and others) can do to fight it. However, I'll be honest here—I do fear diabetes; however, I use this fear to motivate me, rather than allow it to immobilize me.

Here is my manifesto:

- I will stay open to hope. Hope for a better life for the generations that follow me, hope for a cure, hope that complications stay at bay.

- I will fight ignorance and attempt to educate people when I would rather fly into a rage, saying, "I have had diabetes for 37 years! Do you really think you have the right, or even the knowledge, to question me about a glass of wine I am about to consume?"

- I will refuse to listen to "cause-and-effect" judgments about this disease that have not been proven.

- I will always take time for a newly diagnosed person and his or her family.

- I will do my best to manage what is within *my* control and will try to tolerate the fact that much is not.

- I will surround myself with people who bring humor to every situation.

- I will not sacrifice my life to diabetes. It is just a disease, after all.

The Bigger Picture

You also have things that you will do to navigate your own road with diabetes. It is a journey that none of us signed up for, but that we find ourselves taking nonetheless. So let's think about this strategically, both as individuals and as a group. What can we do to make the hard parts easier and the good parts last longer? How can we make sure that our actions not only help us, but also make a difference for those who have similar challenges? What can we do to make our efforts "stick" longer?

I've presented my ideas in the book to give you not only some guidance in "getting to better" in your own life, but also some reassurance that you are not alone in this thing. There are others out there—many of us. Our efforts can be synergistic—if we can figure this out, we can be a mighty force to bring long-needed changes to our world, whether the result is better information about diabetes in the world, a cultural change to remove the guilt and the shame that surrounds our disease, or the President putting his pen to a new piece of legislation that may help people living with diabetes. We can make these things happen. Don't doubt it for a minute.

A Word from Coauthor Julie Stachowiak

Let me start by saying that I do not have diabetes. I do not know what it is to live with diabetes, besides a 4-month "dance" with gestational diabetes during my twin pregnancy, which really doesn't count. However, that experience gave me the tiniest bit of insight on what it is like to test my blood glucose four times a day, often getting results that left me scratching my head, despite my best efforts to "do the right thing."

What I do know is what it is like to live with a different chronic disease, multiple sclerosis (MS). I know lots about living with MS, including how it can rob you of so much that we all take for granted before we are diagnosed with something that we will have forever. It was my firsthand experience, as well as what I heard from my readers of the MS site at About.com (http://ms.about.com) that inspired me to write *The Multiple Sclerosis Manifesto: Action .o Take, Principles to Live By*.

See, I had a problem with all the stuff I read about MS. Few of the books I found about MS described life with MS as I was living it. They either contained cold descriptions and statistical probabilities of various disabling symptoms that might come my way, or were filled with vague optimism that did not ring true. I decided to share with other people with MS what it was really like for another real person living with the same disease, and give them some of ideas for what helped me stay afloat on a daily basis and live a life where I wasn't always scared of my disease—a life of dignity.

My friend Lynn and I bonded over our realities living with these diseases, as well as the very special kind of black humor that can make personal stories about self-injecting and humiliating symptoms downright hilarious to people in the "chronic" club. I heard Lynn mention more than once that people with diabetes needed a call to action and concrete strategies for living life, rather than empty promises and constant judgment for failing to meet impossible goals.

We decided to join forces and bring another manifesto, *The Diabetes Manifesto*, to life. Much of the technical stuff was my department, as I am an epidemiologist, accustomed to decoding medical terminology and dry peer-reviewed articles. However, despite what some of the great scientific minds (including mine) would have said about diabetes in these pages, Lynn was quick to shine the "reality light" into all corners and say, "No. I don't think it is that way—in fact, not at all," if she perceived the least bit of judgment or wrongly assigned blame being directed at people living with diabetes.

I have been humbled by my experience working on this book, my experience working with Lynn, and my experience turning ideas about diabetes into actionable strategies for living a better life. I am proud to have participated in this project and it is my sincere hope that you will find something in these pages that dispels harmful notions that your diabetes in any way stands in the way of the person that you really are.

1

Proceed With Confidence

I can confidently state that none of us want to have diabetes. I don't—given the chance, I would erase this disease from my life completely.

But, I can't. Unfortunately, with the exception of those people who have immediate plans to get pancreas transplants, we are pretty much all stuck with it.

Because diabetes is not really the type of disease that we should forget about until it "acts up," we have to figure out what role it is going to play in our lives. Some people make diabetes the headliner. I have met many of these people over the years through my work and in other situations. You may know some of them—all they seem to be able to talk about is diabetes—a delicious gourmet dinner set in front of them becomes a plate of carb counts, a vacation to an exotic locale is described as a detailed account of the challenges of managing blood glucose in a foreign setting, with no mention of culture or scenery. It's "all diabetes, all the time" with these people. To be honest, I find this extremely boring. To be really honest, I avoid these people like the plague.

Then you have the people on the opposite end of the spectrum who refuse to let diabetes in at all. They try to ignore it, hoping it will go away. It never does. Maybe this denial occurs because people live in fear of this disease and what it can do. They hear the judgment coming at them from all sides and may believe (consciously or subconsciously), that they brought diabetes (particularly type 2) upon themselves and that every small challenge with high blood glucose readings or bigger problem in the form of a complication is their fault, a result of their inadequacy. Shame and guilt are by-products of this.

1

Any confidence needed to deal with diabetes is eroded. They try to hide their actions, their test results, their fears. As they continue to keep aspects of their health hidden, it is impossible to do what needs to be done to manage this disease. Without support or confidence, their fears and lack of belief in themselves lead to the self-fulfilling prophecy or wilder blood glucose swings or new complications, and their diabetes gains the advantage.

Take Charge

You are in charge of how you react to your diabetes.

So, given the above examples, what do *we* do with this diabetes component of our identities? We can take a number of paths. We can be people with diabetes who "didn't deserve it," who had brilliant careers as [fill in the blank] cut short, who struggle every day with thoughts of what might have been. We can be defined by our complications, angry when they interfere with our lives and terrified about how much worse they might get. We can compare ourselves to others who don't live with a chronic illness and wonder why it was us, of all people, who have to factor the unknowns of diabetes into our futures. While all of those versions of ourselves might be accurate at different times, we probably don't want them to be included in the vision of who we are striving to be.

For myself, I want to have the courage not to listen to the people who want to tell me (or my mother) that the ups and downs of my disease and my complications are someone's fault—mine, hers, a higher being's, my doctor's. I want to have a strategy for living with diabetes that works for me, that leads me to do what I need to do in different situations—take action at times, sit still at others, get angry—whatever will work to keep me going.

Take Charge

Commit yourself to being the person you want to be.

To do something well, we need to be committed. It needs to be our identity. We need to be convinced that we are or will become who we aspire to be. That conviction is how we get there.

Do Your Best

Build your confidence to attain the dignity, peace, and happiness that you deserve. Be proud of yourself.

This chapter is about confidence. Confidence is a large part of dignity and the inner calm that comes from knowing that you can do this. Confidence is also one of the most difficult things to find and hold on to when living with a changing chronic disease. Ask yourself—how different would your life be if you faced your diabetes with calm assurance and felt in control, not of your blood sugars, but of your life? Confidence comes from inside, from always knowing where one is going, even if it changes. It is having an identity that you are proud of, both as a guiding tool for your own actions as well as an image that you present to others.

Develop Your Personal Mission Statement

Mission statements are brief descriptions of the fundamental purpose of a business or organization. These institutions create mission statements to help focus their efforts and prevent things from getting too chaotic when confronted with internal problems or external challenges. Basically, mission statements are designed to keep the company or organization on track so that it can achieve its goals.

For example, the mission statement of the American Diabetes Association states, "Our mission is to prevent and cure diabetes and improve the lives of all people affected by diabetes."

Many people with diabetes are constantly bombarded with "noise" that is destructive—from others, from themselves, or an unexpected result from a glucose monitor can seem to be judging us harshly. Given this, a bigger vision may just be the thing that keeps you focused and determined.

Writing a mission statement for yourself will help you become more determined and focused on what you want to do and who you want to be, as well as define how your diabetes fits into these plans.

Take Charge

To be in control, you need to know where you are going. Create your personal mission statement today.

Here are the steps to writing your own personal mission statement:

Define yourself. The first step of your mission statement is to define who is writing it. You could use your name followed by a description of the roles most important to you, as well as some of the things that you really enjoy.

I'll try out my example on you: *"I, Lynn Crowe, am a dreamer and a 'nudje' (a nuisance) at times. I have a strong opinion of right and wrong. I am a family member, a partner, a friend. I love cooking, wine, music and sarcasm."*

What you put in your statement is up to you—you should include the things that are most essential to your own sense of self.

Write your dedication statement. Next, you will list what you are dedicated to—the things you are trying to accomplish in your life. Your statement defines what you aspire to be. It contains your values and motivates you to stick with your plans.

In my example, I might decide: *"I am dedicated to getting the best of life and laughing as much as possible."*

Do Your Best

Don't just read my personal mission statement. Do one for yourself, and mean it.

Mention your diabetes. Because you have diabetes and it will play some part in your life, it is important to include that in your mission statement. You can write that you "happen to have" diabetes. So my statement continues with, *"I happen to have diabetes."*

Then, put your diabetes in its place. This is where you "lay down the law" to your diabetes. You put limits on your diabetes and how it affects both your role and dedication to living in accord with your values and your goals.

In my case I wrote: *"However, diabetes will take a back seat when it can, so I can keep the fun people up front."*

State your strategy. You can then outline what actions you are going to take to become the person who you aspire to be, as well as how you are going to apply your personal ideals and ethics to living your life. This is especially important for those times where things are turned upside-down and you are trying to juggle stressful situations. List the actions that you are taking to manage your diabetes and complications to keep your attitude and energy high and to live the life that you desire. Be very specific. The more details you include, the more powerful your mission statement will be. I wrote: *"because I am going to learn more, continue to seek the best treatments, and try to live in the moment when things are in balance and deal with them when diabetes rears its ugly head. I will recognize that I am likely wrong for every time I am right!"*

Put it all together. Putting all of my statements together, I now have the following mission statement: *"I, Lynn Crowe, am a dreamer and a 'nudje' at times, I have a strong opinion of right and wrong. I am a family member, a partner, a friend. I love cooking, wine, music and sarcasm. I am dedicated to getting the best of life and laughing as much as possible. I happen to have diabetes. However, diabetes will take a back seat when it can, so I can keep the fun people up front, because I am going to learn more, continue to seek the best treatments, and try to live in the moment when things are in balance and deal with them when diabetes rears its ugly head. I will recognize that I am likely wrong for every time I am right!"*

Repeat this daily for a week. Writing the mission statement once will probably give you something that is good. However, reviewing your statement and thinking about it daily for a week will create a useful and meaningful mission statement for you. That is your goal. It may sound excessive, but repeat this exercise 7 days in a row. You don't have to spend a lot of time each day, but coming back to your statement 7 times will help you to refine the language and make the statement fit your life perfectly. Just spend 5 or 10 minutes tweaking the language, making sure you include everything and honing the overall message of your mission statement.

Do it your way. Don't worry about grammar. No one is going to read your mission statement—the only person it needs to speak to is you. Feel free to change the format of your mission statement if something else will work better for you. You can add extra statements or put in bullet points. Do anything that works for you when creating your statement.

> ### The Real World
> If you don't know where you want to go in life, no one can help you get there (including yourself).

Stick it on the fridge. When you are finished, place your mission statement in a place where you can see it every day. Be proud of it and link everything you do to making it a reality.

Ask for input (if you want). Your friends and family may be able to help you create the right language and items to include in your mission statement. They can give you feedback on how well it describes you and might think of things that you have left out.

Be realistic. Only include things that you plan to do or have the desire to achieve. This isn't a wish list, but a strategic vision to guide your actions. Your goal should be to strive to make each component in your statement a reality.

Start today. Don't wait. Just jot down notes. Don't worry about editing or putting things in full sentences. Get your wheels turning on this.

Take it further. Turn your mission statement into a plan. Take each of the items and write about how you will achieve them. Make lists of the steps you need to take. Take these lists and prioritize the items. Create for yourself a comprehensive plan to manage your illness and achieve the life you describe in your mission statement.

Now that your personal mission statement defines what you want to do and who you want to be, let's figure out how to make it happen.

Self-efficacy Is Your Best Weapon Against This Disease

Henry Ford is quoted as saying, "Whether you think you can or think you can't, you're right." He was talking about self-efficacy, a person's belief that he or she is able to reach his or her goals. Self-efficacy is a concept that psychologists have studied for decades, which has been linked to successful coping with chronic illness. Self-efficacy comes from different sources. By paying attention to and capitalizing on those situations where we can gain self-efficacy, we can actually create the confidence that is so crucial to getting what we want and need.

Do Your Best

Think you can and you probably will.

Here is the formula to build up a healthy sense of self-efficacy:

Experience repeated success. The most important contributor to a person's self-efficacy is his or her own success. If someone succeeds, especially in situations where he has had to overcome fear or other obstacles, he has greater self-efficacy. An example of this is self-injecting—especially for older people with type 2 diabetes who are starting insulin therapy. Nobody likes to give himself or herself a shot, some people are downright terrified of it, and very few of us have experience doing it before we are prescribed one of these medications. However, once a person works through his distaste, fear, and inexperience to successfully inject himself a couple of times, these feelings of pride and confidence take over and the whole thing gets easier.

The message here is to make it your goal to succeed once at a new challenge. Then have the goal of succeeding again. If you set small, attainable goals like this, your chances of success go up and you can skirt around much of the stress that comes from looking at the I-can't-believe-that-I-have-to-do-this-every-day-for-the-rest-of-my-life big picture.

If you need help getting to those first couple of successes—with injecting or anything else that is difficult for you, such as starting and maintaining an exercise program or testing your blood glucose, look into cognitive behavioral therapy (there are good books on this that may even get you past some personal "obstacles" to success).

Observe "peers" succeed. Another influence on self-efficacy is seeing people similar to yourself succeed. Most of us have seen people in pharmaceutical educational materials inject themselves, usually while smiling and sitting in their perfect kitchens. Many people, understandably, remain unconvinced that it will be easy for them to do this, after checking out these shiny brochures or slick videos.

However, visiting with people in a forum for others with diabetes or going to a support group and listening to others talk about their first injections, the difficulties they faced, but how they kept trying (and succeeding) anyway, will do much more to convince you of your ability to do the same thing. In addition to "modeling" the behavior of successfully injecting, these interactions also have the benefit of providing tips and ideas, based on people's real-life experiences and trial and error. Interactions with others with diabetes in different situations also can be the source of valuable motivation, in the form of "pep talks," also known as social persuasion. Remember this source of fortification as you face the different challenges that pop up in your life with diabetes—others have been there and they can help.

A great example of success comes from summer camps for where kids with type 1 diabetes show other kids how to self-inject—using kid words, talking about feelings in a kid way, addressing kid concerns. When a camper successfully self-injects for the first time, an announcement is made at dinner—all the kids stand on their chairs to applaud and cheer. They do this with such empathy and enthusiasm that I often think an extremely successful program would pair older people moving to insulin therapy with 8-year-old insulin veterans.

Monitor and Adapt Your Reactions to Situations

Our level of self-efficacy is also determined by how we physically and emotionally feel as we tackle challenges and how we interpret these feelings. Many of us can relate to this in terms of how we respond to the results we get from our blood glucose monitors, which often elicit emotional responses if they are different than we expected. A person with high self-efficacy might look at the result for what it is—data to be used to make decisions on what to do next. A person with low self-efficacy, on the other hand, will interpret that number as "proof" that they don't know what they are doing. They will wonder why they are testing at all if the results just make them feel bad about themselves and their doctors will now have concrete evidence that they are "doing things wrong."

These types of responses to different situations can feed into a cycle of positive emotions in the person with high self-efficacy, who will decide that he or she will look at their blood glucose results as a puzzle or challenge to figure out in a strategic way. On the other hand, our person with low self-efficacy can head into a negative emotional spiral, deciding that they will never get the hang of taking care of themselves, eventually leading to the conviction that the diabetes will get the best of them anyway.

That's all well and good, you might say (if you haven't written all of this off as bogus pop psychology), but how does it break down into action? Albert Bandura, the "father" of the theory of self-efficacy defines it as "people's beliefs about their **capabilities** to produce designated levels of **performance** that exercise **influence** over events that affect their lives."

For the sake of illustration, **"influence"** translates into "I have a problem, but it can be solved or mitigated." In other words, one must believe that it is not fate alone, nor cosmic forces of any type, determining the course of events. It implies that, despite the magnitude of the obstacle or problem, a solution exists in the world, which brings us to the **"performance"** in the definition. This is the plan of attack and subsequent measures taken that *will* get us to our solution. The third vital component is yourself. It is not enough to believe that a problem can be solved and have ideas as to how this can be done—you have to be confident that *you* are **capable** of putting the actions into motion and following through until there is some sort of relief or resolution.

Applying these concepts specifically to diabetes, our health depends on us being able to move through our lives without constant judgment (perceived, real or internal) creating distraction and obstacles. There is no place for concepts of "good" or "bad" blood sugar—this gives these numbers too much power, when what they really need to be are pieces of data that we use to take action. We need to believe that we can do what needs to be done—and then we need to do it.

Do Your Best

Believe that you will succeed in everything that you are doing, even when you don't. Then try again.

Eliminate Self-limiting Beliefs

You may have heard about the "placebo effect," which is a phenomenon whereby a treatment (even a sugar pill) has a positive effect on a symptom or illness, mostly because the person taking it believes in it.

Guess what? It works in the opposite way, too. Called the "nocebo effect," if you believe something is bad, that nothing can make you feel better, that a complication is only going to get worse, or that there is no way you will feel good enough to leave the house that day, there is a *very* good likelihood that you are going to be right.

Know Your Stuff

The placebo effect is the response your body has to something that has no known physiological benefit. It represents the power of belief.

Repeated thoughts take on a certainty, meaning that if your brain replays the message "I am sick, I can't do it," pretty soon you'll be completely convinced. Likewise, if you allow your mind to dwell on the "why me?" aspects of diabetes, you'll never get to the "what next?" parts. Self-limiting beliefs are convictions about yourself that get you stuck, but they can be eliminated with a little effort. First, you have to be able to identify your particular self-limiting beliefs and become aware of the times when they are pushing their way into your thoughts. You then have to create more positive beliefs and actively replace your self-limiting thoughts with these. While this might sound like common sense or even a little silly, it actually can prove to be difficult, as you may not realize just how ingrained some of these beliefs are and how much you are defined by them.

Here are the steps to eliminating self-limiting beliefs, with some examples:

Make a list. Take 15 to 30 minutes and make a list of every negative or self-limiting thought and belief that you have about yourself or how your diabetes is making your life difficult. Some examples might be: "I don't have the energy to make change." "I am too overwhelmed." "There is nothing I can do about my diabetes." "I don't have time." "I don't have the resources I need." "I don't understand what is happening in my body." "Why me?" Write one thought per line on a piece of paper. Try to think of as many of these beliefs as you can.

Create a follow-up thought. Next to each thought, you need to create a counterargument to use as a follow-up thought. This statement can often start with a "but," or can simply be another statement about yourself. For example, if your negative thought was "I don't feel well enough to exercise," your counterargument could be "but it might make me feel better, so it is worth a shot. I can always stop if it makes me feel worse."

The Real World

If you can't convince yourself, you'll *never* convince anyone else.

Use the follow-up. Every time you think one of your negative or self-limiting thoughts, always add the follow-up. It might take you some time to catch yourself thinking or saying the negative thoughts, but you will be more aware of them every day. By adding the counterargument, *even if you don't believe it*, you'll be reducing the power of the negative thoughts to influence you. Eventually, they will come less frequently.

Here are some tips for eliminating (or at least reducing your number of) self-limiting beliefs and the power they have over you:

Have faith. This exercise may seem contrived and difficult, but it truly does work. You really can retrain your brain using this technique. It takes some practice and some patience, but it will expand your confidence in yourself.

Make a really good list of your negative and self-limiting beliefs. You may think that you do not have very many of these types of thoughts, but every person has dozens, or even hundreds, of them. Make your list. If you are having trouble thinking of them, pay attention to your thinking as you go through the day—you are sure to find some negative and self-limiting thoughts that are standing in your way.

Recognize that making the counterarguments can be difficult. You may be so convinced of your negative or limiting belief that you can't see any alternative. Don't let yourself off the hook. How would someone you admire deal with the situation? What would your family say about that? What would you like to believe instead? Find a way to counterargue. Your follow-ups can change over time, but don't let one negative belief go by without challenging it.

Of course, when all else fails, feel free to lie to yourself—anything it takes to silence the negative voices.

> ## Do Your Best
>
> Develop a voice inside your head that is always positive and ready to argue with your negative thoughts. You probably already hear the negative voice talking to you loud and clear, it's time to find the positive one.

Have the courage to let go of your limitations. You may have actually grown fond of some of your negative and limiting beliefs, and may have built parts of your personality around them, which means this exercise will be particularly difficult. Stick with it and try not to be afraid of what happens when you let go for a little while. Remember, you don't have to believe the counterarguments, just try to shake things up a little.

Add the counterargument to your speech as well as your thoughts. If you hear yourself telling someone "I just can't figure out what I can eat and what I should do," be sure to follow with a counterargument like, "but I'm going to visit a diabetes educator to learn what I need to know." Don't let yourself make negative statements without challenging them.

Present Yourself (and Your Diabetes) to the World on Your Own Terms

We all have lain awake in bed rewinding and replaying situations and conversations that happened earlier that day (or if it was really bad, that week or month), mentally replacing our awkward or goofy or stupid or nonsensical contributions to the interaction with flawless responses that flowed seamlessly as evidence of our amazing intellect and social dexterity. While we cannot predict when someone is going to spring politics or religion or an esoteric/distasteful/bizarre topic on us, we pretty much know that our diabetes will be the topic of conversation at some point with certain people.

Too often, those of us with diabetes cannot communicate what is happening to us, especially if we are caught off-guard or having a bad day. Of course it is difficult—not only does diabetes affect us on so many levels simultaneously, it can also stir up feelings of anxiety, humiliation, and loneliness that are extremely personal and difficult to both talk about and edit at the same time. This may leave the people around us confused and uncertain, but it also takes a big bite out of our confidence when we are unable to express ourselves in a way that makes us proud of ourselves, rather than second-guessing and replaying what we have said to different people.

I tend to find myself being blunt at times, saying things along the lines of "Yes, I know I look like shit. Unfortunately, I don't look this way because I have been drinking too much or otherwise having excessive fun. I look this way because my gastroparesis has me living on liquids for the past several days and I still feel like heaving."

The Real World

Remember that if you can't express how you are feeling, you shouldn't be surprised if no one understands what is going on. It is vital that you learn how to communicate with those around you.

This is not necessarily about disclosing your diabetes status to others. Preparing yourself to talk about diabetes is more about arming you with materials so that you are in control of a potentially awkward situation and can be confident that you will be ready to present the you that you want the world to see.

Write a 30-second Speech About Your Diabetes

I know a woman who was recently diagnosed with lupus. She is private about her life and really doesn't like to share medical information with many people. Not too long ago, she called me in a sputtering rage. She had just gotten off the phone with a friend with whom she had to cancel some plans, citing "a couple little health problems" as the reason. Her friend didn't merely ask what the problem was, she practically reached through the phone demanding details, saying, "Tell me from the beginning! What is it again? How do you spell it? Did you get a second opinion? Why not!?! Tell me everything!" My friend was angry at her, but more upset with herself, because, as she said, "I wanted to stop talking, but I couldn't. I was so flustered and taken off-guard that I was telling this person everything, including details I don't even share with my husband." We've probably all been there before—situations where we end up dismayed that we disclosed such personal details, while also berating ourselves for becoming a social "victim" of someone's whims.

Preparing a speech about your diabetes may seem like a bizarre exercise, especially if you have been living with diabetes for a while. You may be thinking to yourself that everyone pretty much knows how you are doing. However, think about it for a moment. As for myself, I can do the things that need to be done—monitoring, dosing, figuring out food. Most of the time, this comes automatically and I can even forget that I am doing it. People are amazed at how well I am "handling" my diabetes and when I talk about my diabetes at those times, it comes across as no big deal, which is far from accurate. Then there are times when a symptom of a complication catches me off-guard and I get swept up in the moment. If I were to tell people about my diabetes at one of those moments, they would think that I was completely unable to cope. At work, I am often torn between my desire to keep my emotions/feelings about my diabetes to myself and my desire to share a "teachable moment" to enlighten someone.

There are also certain people to whom I have a more difficult time expressing myself, so I end up doing a poor job of it. Some of these people seem too busy to listen to details; others have their own stories to tell; others I just find downright intimidating, although I would like to communicate with them.

Writing a 30-second "speech" about your diabetes on a sheet of paper is one way to tackle this predicament. Think of this as a way to be polite and tell people exactly how much you care to share, while ending with a natural conclusion. Consider including the following information: what types of complications you are dealing with, how severe your symptoms are at the moment and how they are impacting your life, what you are doing to manage your diabetes, and your attitude toward it.

Here is my sample:

Diabetes varies in how much it impacts me on a daily basis, but is always there to some extent. Some days my diabetes is in check, and except for the things I have to do to tend to it— testing my glucose, giving myself insulin—it doesn't interfere too much. Sometimes it is a nuisance, like when my blood glucose starts getting low during a presentation and I have a hard time continuing, or my glucose spikes during a meeting and my sensor beeps loudly and nonstop. Then there are some days that it really, really sucks to have diabetes, with gastroparesis and exploding blood vessels in my retina being the most intrusive "interruptions" in my day. Then there are the days that bring devastation, like finding out my friend just had her third diabetes-related stroke. I deal with all of this because I have to—some days it is just going through the motions because that is the best I can do, and some days I "fake it," pretending to be okay, or better than okay—maybe because I believe other people need me, but probably it is because I need to convince myself that the worst parts are temporary and I will be okay again soon. Focusing on the "not okay" parts only serve to pull me down further, although I can never completely escape diabetes.

Okay, I timed myself on that speech: 40 seconds. Not bad.

Make sure that you practice your speech a couple of times. What you are aiming for is not rote memorization, but to capture the right feeling and elements that will convey what you want to get across. For me it is important that certain people know that even though I do many of my diabetes-related tasks without much fanfare, it is still there, at times more intrusive than others. I also want them to not think that I am covering something up, but sharing an appropriate amount of information.

Make It Better

Those of us with diabetes cannot truly change things about life with this disease until we can articulate our thoughts and feelings about ourselves, our lives, and our diabetes.

Create more than one 30-second speech if you need to. Clearly, you will have different approaches if you are explaining things to young children in your extended family, a parent of your child's classmate or your cousin. Take some time and think about the tone you want to set when you talk to people about your diabetes. Maybe you are looking for sympathy, maybe you are simply informing people, maybe you are looking for advice, or maybe you want a little of the "Holy shit!" reaction. You can set the appropriate tone.

You can also take this exercise to the next level by finding ways to educate others about your condition. Maybe you will start with friends or family members. Explain what you know, tell people about the realities of managing diabetes, talk about the latest treatments. Make it interesting. Use your communication skills and your life experience to make a difference. Tell your story.

Deal With Some Diabetes FAQs

This is a related exercise to the 30-second speech, in that you are preparing yourself to respond to questions, rather than getting caught like a deer in the headlights when people ask something that probably seems innocent enough to them, but stirs up a whole bunch of emotions in you.

Do Your Best

You will be asked questions, many of which will seem ignorant or insensitive. Decide ahead of time if you want to deal with these questions with quiet, patient grace or to firmly educate your audience—it's up to you, as long as you aren't a victim of the moment.

Sit down with some paper and take some time to list questions people have asked or could ask about diabetes. Depending on how long your list is, you may need to choose the questions that are asked most frequently—these are your FAQs. Write an answer for each question. Decide on the tone and emotional quality that you want to respond with. Make your answers as detailed as you like. You may have different answers to the same question, depending on if it is your spouse, mother, child, or random lady at the grocery store asking it.

Here are some of my favorite FAQs:

- How is your "sugar"?
- Oh, so you have the serious diabetes?
- Aren't you grateful it isn't cancer?
- I hear Mary Tyler Moore is going blind. Will that happen to you someday?

It really helps me to have thought out the answers to these questions. This preparation has actually saved me in the past from reacting emotionally and either lashing out in pure, blind rage or bursting into tears, when I am sure the person asking the question had absolutely no idea that they were hitting a nerve.

The Bottom Line

Whether you just picked up this book on your way home from the appointment where the doctor just confirmed that you have diabetes, or you have been living with diabetes for many years, from now on— every day for the rest of your life—you will have a choice how you will live that day as a person with diabetes.

Do Your Best

Be confident in yourself. Diabetes sucks, but that doesn't mean that we can't do our best. Let go of comparisons to other people (healthy or otherwise) and ask yourself what can be done this day to make things better for you and those you love. Then have the confidence to do those things.

I am not Pollyannaish about having diabetes. I have it too, and know that some things are simply out of our control. I do not know when I will be hypoglycemic or when my gastroparesis will force me to endure a liquid diet (or for how long). I do not know which activities I will be able to do later this afternoon, next month, 2 years from now. I cannot tell you that I will not be scared at times or not get so angry that I snap at those whom I love for no reason besides that they are there when I need a target.

However, I can tell you this—I will not give into diabetes, as corny and tiresome as that may sound. I will cling to the confidence that I can do something. Then I will do it—or at least do the best I can. I will tire-lessly work to control the pieces of diabetes and my life that are under my control. I will not judge myself and I will not allow myself to be judged as I go through life with this disease.

2

Be a Diabetes Expert

You *Must* Understand Your Diabetes

I never expected to know this much about diabetes—of course, I could never have anticipated that I *needed* to know this much to stand a chance of taking care of myself.

After many rocky years as a young person trying to follow seemingly random orders from disinterested physicians—with terrible results, I might add—it became clear that I had to get smart about this disease as a matter of survival. I had to build a team of the best and the brightest health care providers, but I also needed to be informed enough to really assess them and their recommendations. I wanted to make sure that these professionals were smarter than I am, at least about the specific aspect of my diabetes that they were helping me to manage.

I also needed to know enough to be able to challenge my medical team when something from their professional knowledge banks did not fit with what I knew from living with this disease 24/7. In my process of finding my team and advocating for myself, I have left a trail of health care providers who probably do not think too highly of me. That is okay—after all, if I had loved them or trusted their opinions, we would still have a relationship.

In the process of learning about diabetes, along the way I found out a great deal about *my* diabetes. This is crucial. Not only do you need to have your stockpile of workarounds and tricks to make life go a bit more smoothly, but you also need to know where you are unique and how you and your diabetes interact. Most physicians assess laboratory results and proceed with treatment strategies based on a combination of scientific knowledge and clinical experience. An important ingredient in making choices as to what will have the greatest chance of working out is input from the individual. Again, the averages and statistics that physicians rely on are based on a big pile of data taken from lots of people. I am not "lots of people;" however, and neither are you.

If you are one of those people who think "my doctor will tell me when I need to do something different," hear this: That is *not* good enough. As eloquently stated by authors Michael Weiss and Martha Funnel in *The Little Diabetes Book You Need to Read*:

> A diagnosis of diabetes is life-changing. This chronic, unrelenting condition requires attention 24 hours a day, seven days a week. It is always present. Almost everything you eat and do – every minute, every hour, every day – affects your diabetes. The 24/7 intensity is part of what makes diabetes so different from most other diseases.
>
> Yet most people who have diabetes spend no more than an hour or two a year with their healthcare professionals. Who will manage it for the remaining 8,758 hours if not you? That is why the primary responsibility rests with you and not your health care professionals.[1]

For us to do this—to manage our diabetes—we have to know stuff. We have to know what the diabetes is doing to us so that we know why we are taking specific actions. We also need to know if what we are doing is working, or if it is time for a new strategy. This is no small undertaking.

Know Your Stuff

You *must* understand your illness, your symptoms, and your medications if you are going to be in control of your life. There is no other choice.

In the world of public health, there is much discussion of a concept called "health literacy." Health literacy is defined in *Healthy People 2010* as "the degree to which individuals have the capacity to obtain, process, and understand basic health information and services needed to make appropriate health decisions." In most cases, when a deficit of health literacy is discussed, it is in reference to low-literate people or people incapable of making decisions. Many people in these situations are afraid to ask questions, do not fully understand their diagnoses, or are overwhelmed by prescribed treatment regimens or medication side effects; all of which leads to reduced adherence and worsening health.

However, as people with diabetes, the degree of health literacy that we need to attain to meet the above definition goes far beyond being functionally literate and understanding the logistics involved in keeping appointments with a physician. Diabetes is a very complicated disease—a vast jumble of serious complications stirred in with a big mess of confusing glucose levels and treatment options in the case of type 2 diabetes. Living with type 1 diabetes comes with its own set of very different challenges. It is likely that if you visited several physicians, each one would have a different recommendation or toss the options back in your lap for you to choose from. In this circumstance, the health literacy that is required to "make appropriate health decisions" is overwhelming, even considered by many people with diabetes to be out of reach. So they give up.

Know Your Stuff

For those of us with diabetes to be truly health literate, we will pull information from vastly different specialties, depending on our situation. These may include endocrinology, ophthalmology, nephrology, gastroenterology, psychology, clinical trial research, immunology, nutrition, and sometimes even fields like urology and acupuncture. You need to become your own expert; no one else can do it for you.

Not comprehending basic principles of diabetes makes every strange glucose result or symptoms of a potential new complication a surprise, and decisions get scarier. This can emotionally and mentally overwhelm people to the point that they try to shut out everything about their diabetes.

For instance, we not only need to know how to monitor our glucose levels, we need to know *why* we are doing it—what are we going

to do with these results, how are we going to use them to take action
and to make stuff happen?

Here is a typical exchange between a primary care physician and
his patient with type 2 diabetes:

Physician: "Are you testing?"

Patient: "Yes."

Physician: "How are your numbers?"

Patient: "Good."

Physician: "Oh, good, because they were high last time."

Patient: "Yeah."

Physician: "So, it looks like we are doing better now. Great."

Making any sort of decision based on such a vague, nonquantified
answer is unacceptable. Decisions and actions should be motivated by
data. Much of this data comes from us—from our glucose testing logs,
descriptions of hypoglycemia we experienced, reported side effects and
difficulties that we are having with our treatment regimen, and specific
details of symptoms which may point to an emerging complication.

Developing a specific skill set around finding the answers that you
need to discuss things with your physician (calm your nerves or know
what to expect) is essential. An often-overlooked aspect of living with
diabetes is that each person needs to intimately understand his or her
own diabetes to be able to discuss their status with physicians, know
what effects their medications are having, and sense where they are in
terms of well-being and overall control of their blood glucose. How a
person with diabetes "feels" is a complicated combination of symptoms, both intermittent and constant, blood glucose levels, side effects
from medications, and how he or she reacts to and copes with these
physical states.

Besides all of these advantages from knowing your stuff around
diabetes, I want to put in one last plug—being an expert is fun! I can
get some mean-spirited enjoyment out of drilling an arrogant general
practitioner on his knowledge about some of my more esoteric complications in such a way that he would never think to ask me a question
like "how's your sugar?" However, having a solid foundation of knowledge also allows me to have a deeper discussion with my brilliant
endocrinologist and hold my own.

Quick and Dirty Diabetes Facts

Before we even get started on this section, I have to give a disclaimer on the word "facts" in the section header. There are many things about diabetes that are known to be true beyond a reasonable doubt, until proven otherwise. However, there are many more aspects of this disease that escape being pinned down and earning the title of "fact." We don't know with certainty what causes diabetes; we don't know how to cure diabetes; we cannot always predict the prognosis of individual people with diabetes; we don't know when or if a complication will occur; and we can't be sure that a given treatment or regimen is going to work in an individual or for how long it will be effective.

So that leaves us with some stuff that we are pretty sure about, large gaps in knowledge, and a whole bunch of educated guesses. I'm going to do my best to give you the latest thinking on the basic aspects of diabetes, but encourage you to stay curious, question everything, keep looking for information, and remain flexible in your thinking about this disease. Remember, I am not an MD and in no way intend for the information in these pages to substitute a frank discussion with your physician. Again, my goal is just to get you to a basic understanding around some of these concepts so that you can continue to learn about them.

Learning takes effort, often hard work and experimentation in a step-by-step manner. A teenage boy recently explained to me his complicated process for figuring out how to dose his insulin so that he could eat pizza, which presents a bigger challenge than many foods because of the combinations of fats and carbohydrates. He detailed his trial-and-error "pizza project" with pride. It was complex and involved a lot of testing, a lot of research. However, think of the alternative of not learning. Either he would have little control over his blood glucose levels after eating pizza or he would be unable to join his friends when they ate pizza. He chose to learn what he needed to in order to keep up with life.

If a specific concept interests you or you have an inevitable question or doubt about something, do your own research—some guidelines are provided later in this chapter. When investigating a topic, you will probably find that even a very narrow question opens up Pandora's box with different opinions from "experts," as well as from the very people living with diabetes. Don't get discouraged—question what is written here, question your physician, question everything until you feel comfortable with the answer.

What Is Diabetes?

Put simply, diabetes is too much sugar (glucose) circulating in the blood.

This occurs for different reasons and at varying levels of severity, which are described very briefly below.

What Are the Types of Diabetes?

Type 1 Diabetes

Type 1 diabetes is a condition where the body is making *no more insulin* because the cells in the pancreas (called beta cells) that make insulin have been destroyed. This process usually takes some time, months or even years after first symptoms, but there is nothing that can be done to save the cells. It is thought that this is an autoimmune disease, meaning that the body's own immune system mistakenly destroyed the beta cells, rather than recognizing them for the good guys that they are.

Type 2 Diabetes

Type 2 diabetes is characterized by insulin resistance and deficiency. In other words, there is still insulin being produced by the body, but *the body cannot use the insulin properly* or *not enough is made*. This is likely because of a problem initially with the cells themselves, specifically with the insulin receptors on the cell—the insulin receptors are like a lock that opens up to allow glucose to enter and be used for energy when insulin (the key) is present. In the case of type 2 diabetes, the cells are unable to access circulating glucose because of faulty insulin receptors or an inadequate number of insulin receptors on the cell. This problem is made worse when people are overweight or obese (as 80% of people with type 2 diabetes are), as many people who are overweight have fewer insulin receptors on their cells. The body responds to this "insulin resistance" by making more insulin, then more, then even more—until, in many cases, the pancreas simply wears itself out and can't make enough insulin.

Gestational Diabetes

Gestational diabetes occurs in pregnant women. It is thought that in some women (4% of all pregnant women), hormones from the placenta block the ability of the cells to process insulin, creating insulin resistance. Usually, this form of diabetes disappears upon delivery of the baby, but these women remain more likely to develop type 2 diabetes later.

LADA or Type 1.5 Diabetes

LADA stands for latent (or late onset) autoimmune diabetes in adults, but is also referred to as type 1.5 diabetes or double diabetes. This is a relative "newcomer," a hybrid of type 1 and type 2 diabetes that is becoming more prevalent, but that there is no true consensus around. LADA resembles type 1 diabetes—the beta cells of the pancreas are attacked by the immune system and eventually stop making insulin—but is not usually diagnosed until after the age of 30. It is thought by some that LADA is a kind of type 1 diabetes that is very slow to develop.[2]

Prediabetes

Prediabetes is a situation where the blood glucose levels are in limbo—higher than normal, but not high enough for a diagnosis of diabetes. It is often referred to as "insulin resistance," as it indicates that the cells are not using insulin as efficiently to transform glucose into energy that the body can use. Some people with prediabetes are able to prevent or delay progression to type 2 diabetes through aggressive lifestyle modification. However, not everyone can prevent diabetes 2 from developing, as there are many factors besides diet and exercise that contribute to an individual's course of progression. New research is exploring the use of some diabetes drugs to treat prediabetes in an effort to delay or prevent diabetes, but this is not routine practice at this time.

What Causes Diabetes?

Type 1 diabetes is an autoimmune disease, meaning that for some reason the immune system decided to attack the pancreas and destroy the beta cells that produce insulin. Other examples of autoimmune diseases are Hashimoto disease (the immune system destroys the thyroid gland) and multiple sclerosis (immune cells attack the myelin covering on nerves in the brain and spinal cord). It is hard to say why this happens in some people. There is some genetic factor, but this is not enough to directly "cause" diabetes by itself. In fact, although about 10% of the people carry the gene for type 1 diabetes, only about 1% of the population actually develop it.

Like other autoimmune diseases, most likely there is a chain of events that happens—when all these factors line up "just right," certain immune cells go rogue and attack. No one knows exactly what the necessary components are, but it is likely that if a person has the "right" genes for diabetes (which happens to be more common in certain ethnic groups) and gets infected with a certain virus or bacteria, this causes their immune system to ramp up to fight the illness. In the process, there is an imbalance, and the components of the immune system that are supposed to hold each other in delicate check fail to perform, so some specific excited immune cells hone in on something besides the infection—the beta cells in the pancreas, incorrectly recognizing them as foreign and working to destroy them all. A recent study points to a defect in the human leukocyte antigen region of the genome (the part of the immune system that helps T cells figure out if something is foreign and should be attacked by the immune system), which basically causes the T cells to overreact and identify a person's own cells as dangerous invaders.[3]

Type 2 diabetes is a different story. Type 2 diabetes happens when the body's cells become resistant to insulin or the pancreas slows down insulin production. Insulin production in this case is not affected by the beta cells being attacked by the immune system—instead, the beta cells just get "worn out" from overuse, trying to keep up with high glucose levels and the body's growing demands for insulin. In fact, it looks like beta cells actually die through a process called "apoptosis," and most people with type 2 diabetes have 40% to 60% less beta cells by volume than people without diabetes.[4]

There is a very strong genetic factor at work in type 2 diabetes, meaning that people with close relatives with type 2 diabetes have a much higher chance for developing it. For instance, if one parent has type 2 diabetes, each child has about a 15% to 25% chance of developing it, depending on when the parent was diagnosed. If both parents have type 2 diabetes, there is about a 1 in 2 chance that their child will develop it. Again, no one can determine with certainty the direct causes of type 2 diabetes, but it is much more complicated than the common assumption that "eating too much sugar" is the culprit. Although lifestyle factors like poor diet and inactivity seem to be important components, they may be the ingredients that trigger diabetes in people who are genetically predisposed to type 2 diabetes, rather than the direct cause.

We do know that excess body fat increases insulin resistance, which often contributes to developing diabetes. This is because there are fewer insulin receptors on fat cells than on muscle cells, meaning that these cells have fewer places for insulin to bind to, limiting the cell's ability to use the glucose in the bloodstream. In addition, fat cells release free fatty acids, which also interfere with glucose metabolism. This is a vicious cycle, as the glucose that is not metabolized by the body for energy is stored as fat, making more fat cells. An estimated 80% of people with type 2 diabetes are overweight or obese.[5]

Other factors which could play a role in "causing" or contributing to type 2 diabetes include (although there is not complete agreement on some of these factors): chronic stress, having a low birth weight, being older than the age of 65. Although stress releases hormones that make it more difficult for insulin to work, in people with normally functioning insulin receptors this is usually not a problem. When people say that a stressful event "caused" their diabetes, they probably already were insulin resistant and an extreme circumstance just revealed the fact that there was not enough insulin or their cells are not able to use available insulin efficiently.[6]

Interestingly, although people who smoke have a higher rate of developing type 2 diabetes than people who never smoked, when people quit smoking, their risk for developing type 2 diabetes is higher within 3 years of quitting, returning to the same level as "never smokers" after 10 years. Some experts think part of this excess risk might be related to weight gain that is often seen when people quit smoking.[7]

Other Causes of Diabetes

There are other kinds of diabetes, meaning that there are many other causes for high blood glucose levels, such as infections, hormone imbalances, genetic syndromes, and exposure to certain chemicals. Some of them are reversible and blood glucose levels will return to normal after the direct cause is eliminated, such as acute pancreatitis or taking medications that reduce insulin action, like corticosteroids. Some causes can result in diabetes that is controlled with pills, whereas others result in diabetes that requires insulin.[8]

How Common Is Diabetes and Who Gets It?

Experts think that 220 million people in the world are living with diabetes. In the United States, it is estimated that about 24 million people have diabetes, 3 million of whom have type 1 diabetes, with the vast majority of people living with type 2 diabetes.[9] However, only 75% of them have been diagnosed, leaving an estimated 3 million people who are unaware that they have diabetes. It is also thought that 57 million people in the United States have prediabetes.

Risk Factors for Diabetes

Although most of you who are reading this book have already been diagnosed with diabetes, some of you may have been told that you have "prediabetes" or are insulin resistant, and now you are worried. Some of you may have relatives with diabetes and are aware of the genetic link that increases your risk for diabetes—you may want to know what your risk profile looks like and how you should monitor your situation in regard to diabetes.

For different reasons, people often wonder if they should be worried about developing diabetes. Although I wouldn't recommend that anybody engage in active "worry" about diabetes, I do think that people meeting any of the following characteristics follow the recommendations of the American Diabetes Association and get tested, using one of the tests described below (usually the fasting plasma glucose test is the most readily available), repeating the test at least every 3 years if the results were normal, or more frequently if you have several risk factors. If you have been told that you have prediabetes (impaired glucose tolerance, insulin resistance, and fasting blood glucose is between 100 and 125), you should get tested yearly. Everyone older than 45 years old should also be tested.

You are at higher risk for diabetes if you:

- Have a close relative (parent or sibling) with diabetes
- Are of a certain ethnic background (African American, Asian American, Latino, Pacific Islander, Native American, or Alaskan Native)
- Are overweight or obese
- Have certain lifestyle factors, like physical inactivity, smoking, high-fat diet, and consumption of large amounts of alcohol

- Have high blood pressure (140/90) or are taking medicine for high blood pressure
- Have a history of cardiovascular disease
- Have low HDL cholesterol (below 35 mg/dL)
- Have high triglyceride levels (above 250 mg/dL)
- Have tested in the prediabetes level before
- Have polycystic ovary syndrome
- Have given birth to a baby weighing more than 9 lb or were diagnosed with gestational diabetes

How Is Diabetes Diagnosed?

Diabetes is diagnosed with blood tests that detect the amount of glucose circulating in the blood. Unlike many other chronic diseases, the diabetes diagnosis is pretty straightforward—you either have it or you don't. There is really no such thing as "a little bit of sugar" once blood tests show that your blood glucose levels are above a certain level. (An exception to this may be a test result that shows blood glucose within a couple of points of the cutoff for a diagnosis of diabetes—in some cases, people are able to adopt aggressive lifestyle changes or lose a significant amount of weight and drop these numbers back into the "prediabetes" category. These people should have their blood glucose monitored yearly. The other exception is gestational diabetes, as blood glucose levels usually return to normal in women with gestational diabetes once they deliver their babies.)

In most cases, a diagnosis of diabetes will not be made on the basis of the results of one test. Rather, the physician will want to repeat the test to make sure that the results are consistent before telling you anything very concrete or starting treatment. Exceptions to this are blood glucose levels that are very high or elevated glucose levels in a person with symptoms of diabetes, as these people may need more urgent treatment to stabilize blood sugar to prevent acute problems.

Also, physicians usually don't hesitate to make a diagnosis of gestational diabetes following the oral glucose tolerance test, as they tend to err on the side of caution with this one and recommend that pregnant women implement certain dietary changes and home monitoring.

Fasting Plasma Glucose Test

As the name implies, this test determines the amount of glucose in a person's blood after they have fasted (not eaten anything) for at least 8 hours. Because this test requires fasting for 8 hours, it is a good idea to schedule your blood draw for first thing in the morning and bring a snack with you to eat afterward. It is also important not to drink coffee or diet cola before your test, as caffeine causes blood sugar to rise.

Results (mg/dL glucose in the blood) indicate the following:

- 99 or below = normal
- 100 to 125 = prediabetes
- 126 or higher = diabetes

Oral Glucose Tolerance Test

The oral glucose tolerance test is used when a person has normal or borderline fasting plasma glucose levels, but has risk factors for diabetes (or is pregnant) and additional testing is needed to definitively rule out diabetes as a possibility. It may also be used to diagnose prediabetes.

This test also requires fasting for 8 hours, then drinking a special beverage containing 75 g of glucose and having blood drawn later to see how efficiently the body processes the glucose in the beverage. If the person is not pregnant, there is usually one baseline blood draw (before drinking the beverage) and another draw after waiting for 2 hours.

When this test is used to test for gestational diabetes, the beverage contains slightly more sugar (100 g) and there are 4 blood draws: at baseline, after 1 hour, after 2 hours and after 3 hours.

This test should also be scheduled for first thing in the morning because of the fasting issue. Bring along a book to distract you for the hours that you are waiting for the next blood draw(s). The real discomfort (in my opinion) associated with this test is the nastiness of the beverage that you have to drink. You are often given a choice of flavors (I once heard to always go for the fruit punch) and have to drink this gross-tasting liquid within a 5-minute period. Don't be surprised if you feel slightly nauseated after the drink.

Results (mg/dL glucose in the blood) after 2 hours in a nonpregnant person indicate the following:

- 139 or below = normal
- 140 to 199 = prediabetes
- 200 or higher = diabetes

Results (mg/dL glucose in the blood) in a pregnant woman that indicate gestational diabetes are as follows:

- Baseline/fasting = 95 or higher
- After 1 hour = 180 or higher
- After 2 hours = 155 or higher
- After 3 hours = 140 or higher

Random Plasma Glucose Test

The name pretty much says it all—blood is drawn randomly, meaning it doesn't matter when the person last ate. This test is usually conducted in people complaining of certain symptoms that may indicate diabetes, such as excessive thirst, urination or unexplained weight loss. It is also called the "casual plasma glucose test."

Here, the results are pretty straightforward. A person without diabetes is unlikely to ever have blood glucose higher than 160 mg/dL. Therefore, if the blood glucose level is 200 mg/dL or higher and combined with certain symptoms, such as increased thirst or urination, unexplained weight loss, sores that are slow to heal, fatigue or blurred vision, then the person likely has diabetes. A diagnosis of diabetes will probably not be made, however, until either or both of the other tests mentioned above are run and repeated.

A1c

Until very recently, the A1c test was used by physicians and patients with diabetes to get an information about blood glucose levels in the 2 to 3 months leading up to the test. In early 2010, experts announced that results of the A1c test could be used to diagnose diabetes.

The A1c (or HbA1c) test measures the percentage of glycated hemoglobin in your blood. Glycated hemoglobin forms when glucose molecules attach to hemoglobin (the protein in red blood cells that carries oxygen and gives it the red pigment). Once glycated hemoglobin forms, it is there for rest of the life of the red blood cell, so looking at the amount of glycated hemoglobin gives a good picture of how much glucose the red blood cell has been exposed to during its 120-day life span.

Using the A1c test, a diagnosis of diabetes will be made when the A1c level is greater than or equal to 6.5%. A normal A1c for a person without diabetes is between 4% and 6%.

Other Tests

The following tests are not used to diagnose diabetes per se, but may be ordered when physicians are not sure if someone has type 1 or type 2 diabetes, or if they are trying to figure out the best treatment approach.

C-peptide. The body makes the same amount of C-peptide and insulin. Therefore, by measuring the C-peptide, it is possible to see how much insulin a person's pancreas is making. This can be useful to determine if a person is making very little insulin, or if they are making enough insulin, but their cells are resistant to the insulin. This information will help the physician decide what kind of treatment to try. This test is usually performed in people with type 2 diabetes, but is also used in people newly diagnosed with type 1 diabetes to determine "residual beta cell function."

ICA/GADA. Islet cell antibodies (ICA) and glutamic acid decarboxylase 65 antibodies (GADA) are "autoantibodies," which attack proteins on the beta cells of the pancreas that produce insulin. The presence of these antibodies in someone who has been diagnosed with diabetes helps physicians to determine if people have type 1 diabetes or (if they are absent) have type 2 diabetes.

A minority of people with type 2 diabetes also have elevated levels of ICA and GADA, as do people with LADA (type 1.5 diabetes). Most of these people with type 2 and all of the people with LADA will eventually need supplemental insulin. GADA tests also are used to screen siblings of people with type 1 diabetes, as these antibodies are often elevated before the person has any symptoms of diabetes.

How is Diabetes Monitored Once a Diagnosis is Made?

The amount of diabetes monitoring varies according to the type of diabetes a person has, as well as treatment goals, type of treatment, and ease of glucose control. It also has a great deal to do with your specific physician and what kind of patient you are.

Some people with early type 2 diabetes will take an oral medication or manage their diabetes with lifestyle changes, only needing an A1c test twice a year. On the other end of the spectrum are the people that must test their blood glucose several times a day to figure out when and how much insulin to inject, working this around the type and quantity of food they are going to eat and how much physical activity they are going to engage in. Then they must test again in 3 or 4 hours to see if they got it right last time and decide what they need to do for the next part of their day.

Collect Your Data—and Then Use It

Before discussing specifics of how, when, and how often people monitor their blood glucose levels, I want to say that I am a huge fan of checking blood glucose and keeping a logbook, regardless of how easily someone controls their blood glucose or what type of diabetes he or she has. I think it is the one thing that we have in our arsenal to help us know when and how to take action, both in the immediate future and in the long term. It shows us how things are going on a very objective level. Without having this data, it is like driving a car without being able to look in the mirrors—you might be on a busy highway or a quiet country road (to continue the analogy) in terms of your chances for an accident, but checking those mirrors frequently will often give you the warning that you need to avoid a little problem or a bigger "situation."

It is not just enough to go through the motions, however—you must also understand *why* you are doing this at all. You need to use this information to make adjustments, to fuel questions, to take action. Some necessary changes will be revealed only after collecting information for days and looking for patterns in your logbook (such as adjusting meds during certain days of your menstrual cycle), whereas other things will be in response to a single reading (such as eating a snack to prevent hypoglycemia). The other part of this picture is the A1c test, which is crucial to knowing the big picture. You *must* insist that this test is done and you need to know the number—if your physician is not doing an A1c test *and* discussing your results with you, then find another physician.

It is also important to me that each of you understand what these tests and checks are *not* for—these results, in and of themselves, are nonjudgmental. They are quantitative data to be used to figure out how to move forward productively. Do *not* allow any result to convince you that you are not doing a good job, that you have been "naughty," that anything that you are feeling is your fault—using your results in this way is simply counterproductive. Stirring negative emotions into our glucose testing sets us up for failure with unexplained high readings or feelings of guilt if we have a pretty good idea why it might be high (we veered from our treatment plan, for instance). Instead of wrapping ourselves in useless feelings of shame, we need to move forward with resolve to figure out the puzzle. If your physician uses value-loaded words like "bad" and "good" when delivering test results, remind him that the only "bad" A1c test is the one that isn't done; tell him that you are ready to strategize to get the results closer to your goals.

A1c

As mentioned above, A1c gives a better picture of overall glucose control and levels than a single measure of blood glucose level taken at one time. For the sake of analogy, I am sure that there are snapshots of you taken at a point in time that shows that you were happy or sad at the minute they were taken—these may differ greatly from a video that covered the last 60 to 90 days of your life, which captured a spectrum of emotion and reveals your predominant emotional state during that time period.

The A1c test is usually performed in a laboratory, although there is now at least one device (A1cNow SELFCHECK by Bayer) that people can use to check their A1c levels at home. Although it is ideal to get your A1c levels checked by your physician (so that fruitful discussion about the results can occur), some people like to have the option to check their own levels between visits to the physician.

The recommendations for frequency of A1c testing are as follows:

- Quarterly (4 times a year)—If you have type 1 diabetes, or have type 2 diabetes and use insulin, have changed medications or are having trouble controlling your blood glucose
- Every 6 months—If your blood glucose seems stable (consistently within target range) and you are adherent to your medications and meeting other goals
- As needed—If your physician is trying to optimize your therapy, or if you have other goals, like pregnancy, where an optimal A1c is very important

However, you and your physician may want to run the test more frequently than this. Many physicians like to test any of their patients who use insulin 3 or 4 times a year as a matter of routine. Some physicians may also want to test patients whom they suspect may not be adherent to their treatment, who complain of certain symptoms, or who do not monitor their blood glucose levels frequently. It is more likely that every physician will order an initial A1c when they diagnose someone with diabetes or when they get a new patient with diabetes, to establish a baseline of effectiveness of any treatment plan that is decided on. Let me reiterate what I wrote at the beginning of this chapter: Checking your A1c levels is an important part of managing diabetes. If your physician isn't ordering this test (and discussing the results with you) . . . *ask* him or her to do so or find another physician.

The recommendation of the American Diabetes Association is to aim for an A1c of around 7% or a little lower for *most* people, although certain populations, like children and people with specific complications, may have different goals. Although it is usually not recommended to go for much lower than that for most people, as this can result in more frequent or severe hypoglycemia, the American Association of Clinical Endocrinologists urges that people strive for an A1c of 6.5%, which members claim is very achievable through "persistent titration of appropriate therapies"—in other words, early use of insulin and frequently adjusting dosages.[10]

I think the wisest recommendation is for you and your physician to work together to find the tightest glucose control strategy that can be followed without overly frequent or severe hypoglycemia. This will be a matter of trial and error and will depend not only on your efforts, but also on how your body reacts to your treatment strategy.

Some people are curious as to why A1c cannot replace home blood glucose monitoring. You have to remember here that the A1c is an *average* of what has been happening with your blood glucose levels over the past couple of months. Therefore, although you expect to see an A1c of 7% (equaling an average blood glucose of 147 mg/dL) in someone whose blood glucose stays in a pretty tight range of 120 to 160, you could also get an A1c of 7% in someone whose blood glucose is all over the place, with severe hypoglycemic lows of 40 and highs above 300, as long as they average out to 147. However, one person will probably feel significantly better than the other.

Estimated Average Glucose

The estimated average glucose (eAG) is basically a different way to state the results of the A1c test, which uses the same units as a glucose meter (mg/dL). The thinking is that it will be easier for people to understand A1c results reported in this way. The American Diabetes Association has a converter at http://professional.diabetes.org/GlucoseCalculator.aspx.

A1c measurements correspond to the following blood glucose levels:

Estimated Average Glucose/eAG (mg/dL)	A1c (%)
126 mg/dL	6
154 mg/dL	7
183 mg/dL	8
212 mg/dL	9
240 mg/dL	10
269 mg/dL	11

Self-monitoring of Blood Glucose

More than any other illness, many cases of diabetes rely on the active day-to-day participation of the individual to have the best chance of a good outcome. A powerful tool in this is home blood glucose monitoring.

The vast majority of people who monitor their blood glucose use a small meter that can deliver results within 10 seconds after a tiny amount of blood is deposited on a test strip. There are all sorts of features available: meters can store information over a long period of time, and some allow you to download this data to a computer program, chart these results, and average these results. The meters vary in speed, size, amount of data they can store, and how much blood is needed for a reading. There are also differences in price and how much the test strips cost. All of these meters can use blood from a fingertip, but some of the newer ones can use blood from other sites, like the forearm or palm of hand (although results from these samples may have to be interpreted differently).

How frequently you measure your blood glucose depends on what you and your physician agree on and will be different for different people. For instance, people with type 1 diabetes will probably be told to measure their blood glucose at least 3 times a day (this may be before meals, after meals, and at bedtime, depending on what their situation is and what kind of insulin they are using), but more people monitor 6 to 8 times a day. Pregnant women with preexisting diabetes may eventually be testing their blood glucose levels as many as 6 to 10 times a day in the third trimester and women with gestational diabetes will test around 4 times a day until they deliver.

For people with type 2 diabetes, the recommendations are not really clear-cut. If you have type 2 diabetes and are using insulin to control your blood glucose, you might want to check a couple times a day, depending on the type of insulin used and the frequency of dosing. However, there seems to be difference of opinion about blood glucose testing in people with type 2 diabetes who are not taking insulin (meaning those either taking noninsulin medications or working to control their blood sugar through dietary measures). Depending on your physician, your treatment plan, and your A1c test, among other factors, you may be told to monitor your blood glucose levels once a day or more at specific times to see how you are responding to treatment. You may be told that home blood glucose testing is completely unnecessary and not to worry about it. You may also be instructed to learn how to use a meter and to test your blood glucose anytime you are feeling strange, to ensure that your blood glucose is not dangerously low or high.[11]

Regardless of the type of diabetes that you have or the type of medication that you are on, you may also want to check your blood glucose more frequently when you are trying to figure out how something affects your blood glucose. For instance, you may be trying a new form of exercise or exercising at a greater intensity. You may want to take a close look at what happens to your blood glucose with a new medication or when you try different kinds of foods. You may want to see if you are one of those women whose blood sugar is affected by premenstrual syndrome (PMS). In each of these cases, you would have different testing strategies—in the case of a certain food, you would want to check before you eat the food, then 1, 2, 3 and 4 hours afterward, repeating the test on another day to really be sure. With exercise, you would test before starting, during (if longer than 1 hour), immediately after, and once per hour for the next 4 hours, repeating the whole experiment on a different day to really see what is going on. If you are trying to figure out how your diabetes may be affected by PMS, you may need to test in the morning at the same time over a couple of months before a clear picture emerges.

The whole idea here is to make blood glucose monitoring work for you—to make it your main source of data to help you make decisions, rather than relying on vague ideas of how you feel or what you think you should do. Remember, most people feel the same physically when their blood glucose is anywhere in the range of 80 to 200 mg/dL, so gauging by how you feel does not really provide good guidance. Make sure that you record the results of your testing so that you can compare them from one day to the next and ask your physician about them if you have questions.

There may also be specific circumstances where the physician or you want to measure more frequently, for instance, if you are sick or trying a new drug or on a medication that is known to raise blood glucose, like corticosteroids. Again, regardless of diabetes type, if you experience hypoglycemic symptoms or otherwise feel strange, it is always good to measure your blood glucose.

Physicians will typically try to strike a balance with frequency of blood glucose monitoring—especially if you tell them what your goals and concerns are. On one hand, readings can be extremely useful in predicting (and preventing) episodes of hypoglycemia, as well as just keeping blood glucose within a narrow range. However, frequent monitoring has also been shown to lead to depression and feelings of guilt, as well as be an unpleasant inconvenience. If you learn to use your readings to solve puzzles and actively engage in trying to "figure it all out," go ahead and test as much as you like. If you are not getting useful information from these readings, discuss this with your physician—he or she will either help you learn how to interpret the readings (or send you to a class) or decide that maybe you don't need to monitor so often. Of course, for some people, especially people taking insulin, there will be a minimum number of times a day you have to monitor your glucose and this might not be open for discussion.

It is important to know exactly how and when to measure your blood glucose at home. You should also know what to do with the data that you get. The American Diabetes Association recommends that blood glucose levels be between 70 and 130 mg/dL before meals or upon waking, and lower than 180 mg/dL after a meal. The American Association of Clinical Endocrinologists recommendation is slightly lower, with a fasting or preprandial (before eating) level of less than 110 mg/dL and a level of less than 140 mg/dL 2 hours after eating. You and your physician should discuss what numbers you will strive to achieve.

Being realistic, for many people these guidelines are a nice goal, but often lead to frustration on certain days when this kind of glucose control eludes even the best effort. I urge you to make every effort to meet these goals, but don't expect every day to be so rosy. Try not to get too overwhelmed or frustrated in your quest for blood glucose control, as getting stressed out about your numbers will only make it harder to keep trying and keep testing.

Your physician should give you guidelines about when to call in regard to blood glucose results. In general, you should call your physician about high blood glucose levels when they are higher than 180 for more than a week or you get two readings in a row of 300 or more, especially if you don't know how to deal with these numbers on your own.

Blood glucose can also be measured continuously with a device that uses a small sensor inserted right under the skin to measure glucose every 1 to 3 minutes. At this point in time, continuous monitoring is not used long-term by many people, as sensors are replaced every 3–7 days and many people cannot get them covered by insurance unless they are having problems or are on multiple daily injections or using an insulin pump, so the costs can be prohibitive.

For many people, however, there is a certain freedom that comes along with the use of these monitors (especially if you learn how to use your data). In my opinion, one of the biggest advantages is the indication of your blood glucose "trend", often indicated by arrows showing you if your numbers are going up or down. The alarm feature is also a great help—I set mine to indicate if my blood glucose is dropping below 80 or rising above 150. This allows me to take action before I get too far "out of bounds." This feature is especially good for people who don't always feel the symptoms of hypoglycemia or experience hypos in the middle of the night. My continuous glucose monitoring system (CGMS) gives me great peace of mind when I am traveling for business and am alone in hotel rooms so frequently. Although there are certainly some issues to be worked out with these sensors, I truly hope that manufacturers will continue to improve these and insurance companies gain a greater understanding of the value of CGMS.

These devices are used in conjunction with an activities log and food, and are calibrated with results of several traditional finger stick measures. More people are starting to use continuous blood glucose monitoring systems as their primary form of checking their glucose, so this is an interesting area to watch for developments.

In (the unlikely) case I haven't gotten the message across yet, your meter is your friend! The bottom line is that checking your blood glucose is the only way to know what is going on—unless your blood glucose is *very* low or *very* high, you will probably feel the same and be unaware of fluctuations that could be easily addressed.

So. . .

If you don't know if you are feeling a certain way because of diabetes, *check* your blood sugar.

If you want to find out if your meds are working, *check* your blood sugar.

If you want to know the impact of a Boston cream donut, *check* your blood sugar.

If you really want to take charge, understand that this is impossible unless you *check* your blood sugar.

Urine Ketone Testing Strips

Ketones are a by-product that is left when the body breaks down fat for energy, which occurs in people with diabetes when the cells cannot access enough glucose. This happens because there is not enough insulin circulating in the bloodstream. When ketones are present, the condition can quickly progress to diabetic ketoacidosis, which is a medical emergency (see Chapter 3 for a description of this condition).

Testing for ketones is performed by dipping test strips into urine—either directly into the stream or into a sample that you collected in a cup. After 15 seconds, the color on the test strip is compared to a chart to determine the level of ketones in your urine (results range from "trace" to "high" or "large" amounts).

Physicians vary on their recommendations on when to check for ketones, but because ketone strips are easy to use and inexpensive, and ketoacidosis is so dangerous, there is no harm in testing more frequently than your physician may recommend. If you have type 1 diabetes, you should check your ketone levels when you are sick, especially if you are vomiting or have fever, or if your blood sugar is higher than 240 mg/dL. People with type 2 diabetes rarely develop ketoacidosis, including those who take insulin. However, if you have type 2 diabetes, you should check your ketones if you are very sick or you are vomiting, or if your blood sugar level is higher than 300 mg/dL and continues to rise during the day. Pregnant women with preexisting diabetes will probably be directed to test once per day in the morning before eating. Women with gestational diabetes may also be asked to test ketones under specific circumstances.

Ideally, you will have a plan as to when to test for ketones and when you need to call your physician about the results (see Chapter 4). If you do not have such a plan in place, call your physician if you have moderate to large amounts of ketones present.

Monitoring of Complications

Although strategies for monitoring diabetes emphasize checking blood glucose levels on a daily basis, as well as over the longer term, it is crucial that people with diabetes and their physicians be always on the lookout for complications, as well as keeping a close eye on those complications which are already known to be present. This will allow for quick action to lower the risk of developing the complication or slow worsening of the complication.

Your physician should have a plan to monitor different parts of your body and its functions that may be affected by diabetes (see Comprehensive diabetes examination, page 107). However, it is also up to you to be on the lookout for any strange symptom. Report *anything* that seems "off" to your physician immediately. Remember, this extra vigilance and quick response could pay off greatly—never worry that a problem or symptom might seem silly or trivial to a physician. Physicians would much prefer that their patients help them look out for potential problems than wait until it has turned into a more complicated situation that requires more extensive care.

Create (and Become) a Diabetes Encyclopedia

Clearly, there is so much to know about diabetes, as well as so many things that remain unknown, that it is difficult for anyone to have a comprehensive understanding of the whole diabetes universe. Not only is it difficult, but for those of us living with diabetes, it is unnecessary—we need to know the specifics of *our* disease and symptoms. One way to get a handle on the information pertinent to our situation is to compile our own "Diabetes Encyclopedia."

Take Charge

Medical terms have specific meanings. If you use one, you need to know exactly how the physician will understand it. Improper use of a term could lead to unnecessary tests or other misdirected attention.

I bet many of you have done something that I am guilty of, which can have bad consequences. Raise your hand if you have ever sat and nodded while your physician was using a term that you had absolutely no idea what it meant. You might have thought "I'll look it up later" or "I can figure this out from context," but then you leave and completely forget what the term was. I am always amazed when people call me and say, "The doctor said that I had this thing that starts with a 'b'—no, wait, it was a 'p'—hold on, I take it back, it definitely started with a 'b' and he said that it might be serious."

The other side of this is using a term that you don't understand. Many people have dug themselves into holes by referring to something by an improper term, using it because it had the right number of syllables or seemed familiar. My friend's father was famous for doing this, one time announcing at Thanksgiving dinner that he had just been diagnosed with endometriosis, when what he really meant to say was "diverticulitus."

It is important—no, *crucial*—to master the vocabulary, terms and concepts around diabetes. If you listen to a lawyer or a chef talk, there is a special language that efficiently and accurately communicates concepts in their specific field. Diabetes has a language, too—a set of terms and concepts that you need to understand in order to think and communicate well about your illness. If you possess the vocabulary, the world of research also opens up to you, as you begin to navigate ideas around immunology and neurology and decode results of treatment trials.

Here are some steps to mastering diabetes vocabulary and creating a diabetes encyclopedia:

Each day, you will define or explain about five terms or concepts. You can use the Internet or you can refer to books. Once you write out the terms *in your own words* you'll be much closer to understanding and mastering the major concepts around diabetes.

Take Charge

If you can't use a term naturally, in your own words, and explain it to a friend, then you don't yet have mastery of it. Mastery of a term means you are in control of discussions and communications around that topic. It is beneficial to have mastery of at least some of the most relevant terms to your diabetes.

Make a List of Terms to Define

You can keep a running list of terms that you "collect" in your reading about diabetes. Some ideas to get you started are basal insulin, C-peptide, gastroparesis, glucagon, glycemic index, glycogen, A1c, islets of Langerhans, ketones, microalbuminuria. Of course, if you have been living with diabetes for some time, you may already have mastered many of these terms. However, there is always a deeper level of knowledge to strive for, especially if you are interested in following research news. Be sure to include terms specific to your symptoms or situation that you may need when talking to your physician, researching clinical trials or investigating possible treatments.

Schedule Time

You'll need to set aside between 15 and 30 minutes every day for about a week for this exercise. Be sure to schedule this time, otherwise it probably won't happen. You could do it while your family is watching TV in the evening. You could do it over your lunch break at work. It doesn't matter when, but you'll need time to work on the definitions.

Gather Resources

You may have a book or two on diabetes—those often have glossaries in the back that can be really helpful. You may also know a few Web sites that are good (see next section, "Define your questions and get your answers on the Web").

Use Your Own Words

It will be tempting to just look up the words, read the definitions and move on—*Don't do it*. The goal of this whole exercise is for you to have a mastery of these terms. To get that mastery, you need to write them out in your own words. Composing and writing will use more of your brain, which will help you remember the concepts and give you a feeling of expertise and mastery.

You can add to definitions, make them personal and include observations. If you are writing about a symptom you have, you can focus on your level of severity. Make your diabetes encyclopedia about you and focus on the things that are most important to you. Don't worry about format. You don't need to write formal definitions—your entries can be notes, lists, or little sketches. Do whatever will help you remember all the details the best way you can. No one needs to see your diabetes encyclopedia but you, so don't worry about editing and making your entries perfect. Just be sure that you can understand the terms and concepts that you need to know.

Know Your Stuff

Give yourself a little quiz to see if you can answer some questions accurately—for example, How do your medications work? Why do you feel the same hypoglycemia symptoms at different blood glucose levels? Why does high blood glucose make you feel tired?

Try to answer the question "why?" when possible. For example, if you are describing a symptom, try to explain why that symptom occurs. Explain why medications work.

Take your diabetes encyclopedia further by adding more concepts. Include entries on a variety of related subjects that you are particularly interested in, such as, tips to combat side effects from medications you are on, how stress impacts blood glucose levels, or news about stem cell research progress for the treatment of diabetes. Keep making entries in your diabetes encyclopedia as you run across new terms, new treatments and new symptoms.

Define Your Questions and Get Your Answers on the Web

For many people, the Internet has become a surrogate friend to whom intimate secrets are told via blogs, a financial advisor to guide us through rocky investment waters, a place where we can meet all sorts of interesting people (including potential future spouses), and a shopping mall with an infinite variety of goods and services, minus parking lots and crowds. The Internet has also opened up an entire universe of information that, until recently, was only available in medical libraries or stashed away in the brains of researchers and physicians. For those of us with diabetes, the Internet can be a treasure trove of information and options that we used to rely on our physician to transmit to us in annual 20-minute visits. However, much to the dismay of many medical professionals, the Internet has also become a virtual physician to many that seek answers and help, as well as prescriptions, for those who find their way into the "underground."

Do Your Best

Don't surf the Web for medical information without setting up rules for yourself about how to evaluate the things you find. Otherwise your search for information may end up being frustrating and misleading, not to mention overwhelming.

The Internet is wonderful for so many reasons. Some sources can help people navigate confusing situations, calm them down when something unfamiliar happens and provide enough background and support to discuss something new with their physicians in a way that gives them answers. However, the Internet can be not-so-wonderful, and even dangerous. Given the "benefit" of anonymity, anyone can post anything, and, to the casual surfer, completely fabricated diatribes can look just like recommendations based on data coming out of peer-reviewed trials. Often, the more upset or alternative or convinced that people are about something, the more they write about it and the "bigger" it can get on the Internet. Given these potential information "detours" that people can be led down, it helps to have some guidelines in place when looking for answers on the World Wide Web.

In addition, it is very easy to become overwhelmed with the amount or technical nature of the information that can be like a virtual "avalanche" after entering a seemingly simple term or question into a search engine. Following the guidelines below will guide you to appropriate and trustworthy information, but you should also monitor your reaction to the information. Don't try to process all of the information or learn everything there is to know about a topic all at once—read a little at a time, taking breaks to let it soak in and allowing specific questions to form before you go back for more.

Here are some steps for surfing the medical Web:

We Love the NIH

The NIH (National Institutes of Health) is a tremendous institution, and an excellent place to start any health-related search, as many other sites "adapt" their information from the NIH pages. The NIH has compiled information on different diseases and conditions, as well as on all prescription medication, over-the-counter drugs, herbs and supplements, and their uses on a Web site called MedlinePlus (**www.medlineplus.gov**). It sponsors (via Congress) much of the medical research that takes place in the United States. Go there and read about diabetes complications, treatment, financial matters, diagnosis, research, and many other topics. MedlinePlus also has links to other sites like the Mayo Clinic, the American Diabetes Association, the Juvenile Diabetes Research Foundation and the various institutes within the NIH. Although all of the sources found here are reliable, not all of the information is always in total agreement or emphasizes the same things, so definitely read from more than one source when looking for answers.

The Real World

Most people, even many physicians, don't know much about diabetes. You need broad knowledge to assess what you read yourself.

Conduct a Basic Search

When searching for information, there is a fine line between being too specific and not being specific enough. You need to come up with a keyword that an author would have featured prominently in his or her writing. You also need to think about whether your search needs to be specific to diabetes or not. For example, you might find some great suggestions about fatigue from sites about other illnesses. You'll need to keep experimenting and trying to put yourself in the mind of the writer. Generally, you should search using the keyword "diabetes," combined with an additional term that you want information about, such as "numbness."

Read the Address

In your search results, at the bottom of each entry that appears, is the actual address of the site. It will look like this: **www.diabetes.org**. Before clicking on a link, read the address of the site. Look for familiar words from respected places in the address like the following: Harvard, the Mayo Clinic, the Cleveland Clinic, the American Diabetes Association. If an address ends in ".gov," then you can be sure it is a government Web site. If the address ends in ".edu," then you know it is an academic or university Web site. Addresses that end in ".org" are likely to be nonprofit Web sites, but are not always.

Check Your Dates

Pay attention to when an article was written and the last time it was updated. This information is usually at the bottom of the page, but could appear anywhere. Sometimes, dates will not be on Web sites—just do your best to assess when things were written.

Medical Review Matters

Some Web sites will mention that the content was reviewed by a physician or medically reviewed. This means that a physician read through the information on the site and certified that it is correct from a medical standpoint. Look for that, especially when a site is giving medical or treatment advice.

Do Your Best

Be fair when you search. Don't simply search until you find the information that you think you want. Many people use the Internet as a crutch to justify their decisions. Instead, make your searches about finding facts, not opinions that you like or agree with.

Conduct a Site Search

One of the handiest ways to find information is to conduct a site search. In Google, you simply type *site:sitename.com search term* (replacing *sitename.com* with the address of the site you want to search, and replacing *search term* with the keywords that you are interested in). Google will return search results only for that site. For example, if you are interested in information about hypoglycemia from the American Diabetes Association, but don't want to spend a lot of time clicking through links, you could try the following search in Google: *site:www.diabetes.org hypoglycemia*. If you were interested in learning more about a particular medication, such as metformin, from MedlinePlus, you could type the following search into Google: *site:www.medlineplus.gov metformin*. Remember to place a colon after the word *site*, and a space after the Web site address.

Use Google Alerts

This is an extremely handy tool that does much of the "surfing" for you. Google Alerts will send you an e-mail whenever a new Web page appears in the top 20 Web results or top 10 news results for the terms you specify. It's incredibly easy to use—just go to **www.google.com/alerts** and fill out the "Create a Google Alert" form with the search term you are interested in and a couple of other details, like how often you would like to receive the e-mails (I recommend once a day) and your e-mail address. One tip—I recommend putting quotation marks around search terms if they are more than one word, so that an alert on something like "insulin pumps" stays on topic, rather than giving you news on insulin or other types of pumps.

Narrow It Down

Sometimes you have a question about tips to deal with side effects of a medication, a problem related to a symptom that you are experiencing, or something else specific. Go ahead and type in the specific question. Then click on all the links that are returned. Don't worry about where the information is coming from at this point. You'll probably find a forum or a blog where someone with diabetes is writing about the same problem you have. This is good. There are often very helpful suggestions and practical information on these types of sites. You may even find some people to write to and ask directly. Just remember, this may not be medical information, but information from people like you who are trying to deal with their diabetes on a daily basis. That doesn't mean it isn't helpful, just don't do anything drastic without talking to your physician.

Tips for surfing the medical Web:

- Find 5 to 10 really reliable Web sites that you can trust. Start your searches for information there. Make MedlinePlus one of them.

- Find three to five sites written by people with diabetes. They may be blog-type sites or discussion-based sites. Hang out there for a few days and see if there isn't interesting support or information available. Just don't get caught up in people's ranting. When someone is upset about something these days, they write about it and post it to the Internet.

- Don't shop when searching for medical information. You will run across all sorts of ads and products that people are trying to sell you. Assume they are all scams. Don't buy anything. At the very least, be very diligent and check things out thoroughly.

- Stay focused—write down the information you are looking for and try to stick to it, otherwise you could get lost and be spending too much time at the computer.

- Stay on the reliable and trustworthy Web sites at least until you have a mastery of the topics and concepts.

- Read any "worst-case scenario" or "miracle cure" stories with the utmost caution. There are extreme cases of every disease, and diabetes is no exception. These stories are often found on the Internet, as are claims that diabetes is caused or made worse by all sorts of things that we come into contact with every day. Don't let these stories or theories add to your stress or lead you to make extreme changes in your lifestyle without talking to your physician. Do not, under any circumstances, ever change anything about your medication, including stopping it or changing dosages, based on something you read on the Internet (or anywhere else).

The Bottom Line

Based on personal observations, I would guess that about 85% of people, upon receiving a new electronic gadget, tear open the box and start pushing buttons before reading even the first page of the instruction manual. I am notorious for the "figure it out later" approach—I have several electronics that should all work together, controlled by one remote. The pile of remote controls next to the couch is evidence that I haven't gotten around to solving this one yet.

Take Charge

As a person living with diabetes, you simply must put in lots of research and learning time. Knowledge is what will give you as much control over you situation as possible. Knowledge will also make the unknown future much less scary.

We cannot afford to be this way with our bodies, especially those of us living with diabetes. We have to be able to identify what is going on with us to know when to take action and what kind of action needs to be taken. Then we need to be able to talk to our physician about it, so that he has the information that he needs to help us. Only by having some ideas about what it means when certain things are happening to us can we fight the fear of the unknown and create a plan based on knowledge, rather than based solely in emotion.

3

Tackle Complications

Although some of these complications are ugly and the treatments often sound just as unpleasant, I feel it is important to provide information on the potential complications that people with diabetes might face one day to give a jumping off point for personal research, help people recognize the symptoms, and give a brief overview of the available treatments so that people won't rely on scary stories from relatives or the media to form their first opinions of prognosis.

In this chapter, I decided to tell the truth as I see it and have lived it in regard to complications. Many of you will never experience even one of the problems in this chapter, some of you will have one or two to some degree, and a couple of us get to sample many of these complications.

That said, I am now going to say something that many are afraid to: Although you can greatly reduce the likelihood and even the severity of some of these long-term complications, for many people, some will show up anyway. I have read the diabetes books written by doctors that virtually promise that if you do what your doctor says and keep your blood glucose as close to normal as possible, you will *never* have to deal with any of these complications. I guess this makes some doctors and authors feel like they have done their jobs, as they assure themselves that this approach will motivate people to stick to treatment plans (even though research shows that fear-based messages rarely work to motivate people to do anything besides be temporarily concerned). This message also allows these authority figures to be the bearers of good news, as in "yes, you have diabetes, but I can make sure that it doesn't turn into a problem—if you just listen to me." Often, however, the message takes on a negative tone, along the lines of "if you don't do X, then . . ."

This approach does a great deal of harm. It sets people up for failure. It makes people feel guilty if they do experience a complication. It may lead to people ignoring symptoms of complications or avoiding appointments to screen for, diagnose or monitor them, as they are sure that they have done everything right to prevent their occurrence. In addition, for many people with type 2 diabetes, symptoms from a complication may be what led them to the doctor in the first place; therefore, they may be starting off from a place of feeling defeated before they even start to deal with diabetes.

We need to set the story straight, get things right and be proactive, but also realistic and strategic about our diabetes and potential complications. Treatment of diabetes has changed dramatically for the better and this most likely does have a positive impact on the onset of complications. However, there are still many mysteries as to who gets complications, which ones they get, and when they show up. The group that tends to get the attention in books for people with diabetes are those people with relatively tight glucose control and less risk of complications. The people who get ignored in much of the information that is out there are those with either tight glucose control and complications or those with poor control and no complications, as these scenarios don't really fit the prevailing poor blood glucose control equals complications equation.

Given that, here is what I have to say:

- Do what you can to control your blood glucose. It is the one thing in your control that might reduce the risk of developing many of these complications and make the ones you may experience much less of a burden. The problem is that even if blood sugar is a large contributing factor to complications, we still do not have tools that completely mimic how the body functions in someone without diabetes. We need to keep pushing for research to get us closer to perfect. Again, although the news has improved around treatment of diabetes, I still can't give you a guarantee that you will never see one of these things crop up—no one can until we cure this disease.

- Many of these complications are asymptomatic until substantial damage has been done, so it is imperative that you keep appointments to screen for these things, even if you were "perfectly fine" just a year or 6 months ago. In addition, do monitor and react to every possible symptom—no matter how mild or how unlikely you think it might be that you have a particular complication. Catching them early could make a huge difference in how they impact your life.

- Realize that complications are chronic, meaning they don't go away in most cases. Some are constant, while others cause sporadic symptoms that are "on again, off again." However, they can be successfully managed—I am living proof of that.

- Complications are to be respected, but not used to frighten people into behaving a certain way. Fear can immobilize people and if a complication crops up in your life, that is precisely when you need to take action. In fact, by being proactive and strategically monitoring the situation, the action you take in many cases, such as regular retinology exams and foot inspections at home and at the doctor's office, may give you the advantage by helping you catch a complication long before there are any symptoms.

- Again, you can manage your complications—just like you manage your diabetes—however, to do that successfully (in both cases) you have to learn as much as you can. Your tolerance for crappy doctors and unclear treatment strategies must go way down. You must find someone to work with to help you and to give you the tools to help yourself.

Given all that, you can decide for yourself whether you want to read this chapter, skim this chapter, skip this chapter altogether, or just turn to a page featuring a complication that you want to learn more about. Of course, this basic information is not a substitute for your doctor, rather it is a place to check in if you want to get your bearings on a particular symptom you may be having or to help you understand the importance of regular exams and screenings, even in the absence of symptoms, to get an idea on how best to proceed. Also, please be aware that you may have symptoms and/or complications that do not appear on this list that are associated with diabetes. I also want to emphasize again that there will surely be many complications in this chapter that you will never experience.

Acute Symptoms

I encourage all people with diabetes and those close to them (really, anyone reading this book) to at least read through this section on acute symptoms. Hypoglycemia, diabetic ketoacidosis (DKA), and hyperosmolar hyperglycemic nonketotic syndrome (HHNS) can all be dangerous for different reasons. The bright side of this story, however, is that there are pretty objective home tests using glucose monitors and ketone strips that can tell you pretty definitively if there is a problem, so that you can quickly react. Even better, there are easy steps to take to lessen the likelihood that these things will occur or become a much bigger problem. Mark this section for future reference and encourage your people to read it and help you take appropriate action when needed.

Hypoglycemia

Hypoglycemia occurs when your blood glucose gets too low, which causes a stress response in your body. Symptoms, such as sweating or shakiness, come from the release of "fight or flight" hormones, such as adrenaline and norepinephrine. Hypoglycemia is defined as a blood glucose level lower than 70 mg/dL. Many people do not notice symptoms until their blood glucose is lower (and some people never feel symptoms before someone else recognizes them first), although symptoms are felt more acutely and at a higher level during the day when they are wide awake and if blood glucose levels are falling very rapidly.[1]

Hypoglycemia can be influenced by a couple of things, but the basic reason for it is that there is more insulin than glucose floating around in your body. There may be too much insulin in your body because you didn't eat as much or as soon as you anticipated after injecting or the timing of your dosing was too close together. Your blood glucose may also be low because of excess physical activity. Many women experience hypoglycemia at the onset of their period. Or, your blood sugar might just be low because it just is—this disease is *not* always predictable.

No matter how hard you try, if you are on insulin or some of the other drugs, your blood sugar will get too low on occasion, so preparation is crucial. Although hypoglycemia can be scary, and even dangerous, it should not be the reason that you avoid certain medications that will help you control blood glucose.

Although we can (and should) make adjustments to try to avoid these situations, for many of us—including myself—"hypos" happen, despite our best efforts. However, they can be minimized by being vigilant, testing often and constantly tweaking things, based on the data we have.

What Does Hypoglycemia Feel Like and Why Is It Dangerous?

Hypoglycemia can seem kind of benign at the onset, leading people to think that they just might be a little tired and that it can be dealt with at a more convenient time—however, it progresses quickly. As blood glucose falls, judgment and reaction time also become impaired. Symptoms of hypoglycemia include:

- Hunger
- Sweating
- Feeling dizzy or shaky
- Headache
- Pale skin color
- Tingling around the mouth

If blood sugar continues to fall, movements are impaired and can become jerky, you may feel emotionally unstable and you find it hard to pay attention or feel confused.

For some people, especially those who have been living with type 1 diabetes for a while, people who have hypoglycemic unawareness, or people with type 2 diabetes who are on larger doses of insulin, the symptoms may come on much more suddenly (I describe this as "getting slammed") and blood sugar might be lower by the time that symptoms prompt them to check blood glucose levels.[2]

Although it is true that you may have a seizure or pass out if hypoglycemia goes untreated, this is extremely rare and only seems to happen if blood glucose levels are below 60 mg/dL for several hours or if blood glucose drops very quickly.[3] Very few people actually die from the hypoglycemia itself, as we all have a reserve of 200 to 300 grams of glucose stored in our livers in the form of glycogen. Even if someone passes out from hypoglycemia or is hypoglycemic in the middle of the night, this glycogen will be released and eventually the person will wake up. However, hypoglycemia can lead to very serious accidents if it occurs when a person is driving or trying to negotiate stairs.

I will say that there are some pretty excellent videos on YouTube of people describing their experiences with hypoglycemia and how they felt when they were happening. Some of them are actually pretty funny in the way that people use their own words to really paint a picture of their experience, using humor to illustrate sensations that dry, clinical terms just can't get across in the same way.

What Should I Do About Hypoglycemia?

Most people with diabetes learn how to identify the feeling of hypo-glycemia and what to do about it after only a couple of occurrences, but here is the general idea—when you start feeling "weird," here are the steps to take:

1. Check your blood glucose level immediately. Here is yet another instance in which "your meter is your friend."
2. If it is low, treat hypoglycemia with some form of fast-acting glucose, equaling 15 mg of glucose. These can include candy (5–6 pieces, depending on which type of candy), a small amount (1/2 cup) of fruit juice or 3 glucose tablets.
3. Check blood glucose level again 15 to 20 minutes after eating.
4. Repeat if necessary (if blood glucose level is still low and you still feel weird).

The above steps are what we are "supposed to do." However, it is very common for people experiencing hypoglycemia to frantically eat until we feel better, which is usually waaaaay too long and sends our blood sugar rocketing up into the 300s. I remember one situation where my partner asked how bad my hypo had been the night before. I was sur-prised that she knew there had been a problem, as I thought I had been quiet enough so as not to wake her. When I asked her why she thought I had been hypoglycemic, she said that the kitchen was covered with potato chip crumbs. To avoid a repeat of the "eating rampage" scenario, I keep a juice box near my bed. I know exactly the amount of carbs that it contains. This has saved me from dramatic blood sugar surges from "overtreating" my hypoglycemia (and kept my kitchen much cleaner).

Here are some important tips to help us manage hypoglycemia in real-life situations:

- If you aren't able to check your blood glucose levels for some reason, but feel symptoms of hypoglycemia, treat (eat sugar/carbs as above) anyway.

- Plan for hypoglycemia, so that you don't overeat. Make yourself a "hypoglycemia kit" with: 2 portions of your 15 grams of fast-acting carbohydrate measured out; and 2 portions of your 15 gram longer-acting carb measured out. Take this with you everywhere.

- Have a treatment that you know how to use. My daytime treatment of choice is Swedish fish candy—I have been using these for so long that I know exactly how many fish I need to correct my glucose if it is 30 or if it is 65. It is important to have something like this that you really understand, in terms of how much is needed, as opposed to something that you have to figure out how much to take, as it is very hard to really think when your blood sugar is low.

- Have a "nighttime hypo kit" next to the bed containing a bell, a phone, 2 servings of 15 grams of fast-acting glucose and 1 serving of 15 grams of longer-acting glucose, and maybe a glucagon pen. As I mentioned above, I keep a juicebox next to the bed (with the straw already open).

- If you ever test your blood glucose and it is lower than 50 mg/dL, treat yourself for hypoglycemia, even if you don't have any symptoms. It is possible for some people to have hypoglycemia progress to the point of passing out before they have or recognize any symptoms, especially people who have had diabetes for many years or who take certain medications for hypertension or heart conditions. This is sometimes called "hypoglycemia unawareness."

While hypoglycemic unawareness can be a problem, Dr. McCulloch says in his book, *The Diabetes Answer Book: Practical Answers to More than 300 Top Questions*, that although many doctors tell their patients that there is nothing to be done about hypoglycemic unawareness, there may be something to try that could remedy the situation for some people. He says that by making adjustments (in diet and exercise) so that your blood glucose does not drop below 100 mg/dL for at least a week, it is actually possible to regain the ability to recognize symptoms of hypoglycemia, which will allow you to respond much more quickly. I have never tried this myself, but it is worth a try.

For people who know that they have hypoglycemic unawareness and have frequent hypos, a continuous blood glucose monitor (CBGM) might be an option. Bottom line is that frequent testing is key. I see it like driving a car—even though we know accidents can occur, we still drive our cars. However, we take precautions to minimize accidents and harm, such as putting on our seat belts and driving at safe speeds. Hypoglycemia is another place where "an ounce of prevention is worth a pound of cure" and we can reduce problems if we can see them coming.

- Make sure that your people (family, friends, and coworkers) know what to do and not to do if you are having low blood sugar. The things they should understand include:
  - Recognize the symptoms of hypoglycemia (post these somewhere, if necessary).
  - Understand that you may be confused or belligerent if you have low blood sugar and not to trust your judgment.
  - They should know when to call 911 and when to inject glucagon. These discussions aren't fun, but you need to go ahead and have them anyway.
  - Learn how to inject glucagon—a treatment given by injection that stops the symptoms of severe low blood sugar quickly—if needed. They should know where it is (and you should ensure it is not expired). Glucagon is used in extreme circumstances, usually when the person is unable to drink or eat anything themselves (for instance, if you are having a seizure or are unconscious). If they are uncomfortable with this, or you are not confident that they could do it, there are gels that can be smeared inside the mouth that might be easier for them to use.

- ○ They should know not to give you insulin if blood glucose is low.

- ○ Do *not* try to administer food or drinks to you if you pass out.

Many people worry that they could die from hypoglycemia. Although there can be very dramatic symptoms of passing out or even seizures, it is very rare that someone actually dies from low blood sugar. However, hypoglycemia has lead to deaths from automobile accidents. Make a habit of checking your blood sugar before driving (especially if you will be in the car for a long time or in a situation where it will be hard to pull over) or at least checking in with how you are feeling, and do not drive if you feel like you might be at risk of hypoglycemia until you have stabilized your blood sugar.

In my (very strong) opinion, if you are on insulin and any of the above information is new to you, you need to find a new doctor. Your doctor hasn't done his or her job if you are at risk for hypoglycemia and you haven't been given clear instructions on how to deal with the situation. Part of the reason that hypoglycemia can be so scary to some people is that they don't know what to expect from their treatment— this leads people to be too afraid to use their medicines or not know how to use it effectively. I actually heard one person say, "I had no idea that insulin had to be injected until I went to the pharmacy to fill my prescription." What do you think is the likelihood that this person will effectively use their treatment, much less know how to react to hypo- glycemia? We have to demand better instruction from our doctors if we are going to manage this disease and the challenges that crop up.

Different people will be more likely to experience hypoglycemia than others, depending on type of diabetes, medicines they are taking and many other factors. Not all instances of hypoglycemia can be avoided in some people, but getting to know how your medications and other factors work in your body can give you information to reduce the risk of hypoglycemia.

Once again, my motto here is "your meter is your friend." Check your glucose regularly and record the results in a log, making sure that you also note times when you have become hypoglycemic. Study the log for patterns. Review this with your doctor, especially when first learning about diabetes and when trying to figure out your reaction to different things.

Ketoacidosis (DKA)

Ketoacidosis usually occurs in some people with type 1 diabetes, although it can happen to anyone with diabetes. It happens when there is not enough insulin in your body and your cells start burning fat instead of glucose. This can happen for different reasons, for instance, you may be ill and have different insulin needs than usual or you may have missed a dose of insulin. DKA also occurs in people that have diabetes but do not know it, typically in young people with type 1 at the time they are diagnosed. The good news is that, whereas probably close to 100% of kids diagnosed back in my day were in DKA, now only about 30% of kids today are in DKA at diagnosis. This is a huge achievement.

DKA is a very serious condition that can lead to diabetic coma or even death.

What Does Ketoacidosis Feel Like and Why Is It Dangerous?

The initial symptoms of DKA may be fairly subtle and include frequent urination and feeling thirsty. If checked, blood glucose levels will be high (usually above 300 mg/dL), and there will be a high level of ketones in the urine. As ketoacidosis progresses, there will be other symptoms, such as:

- Tiredness and weakness
- Nausea and/or vomiting
- Flushed skin
- Abdominal pain
- Breathing difficulties (breaths will be faster)
- Fruity odor on breath
- Confusion or disorientation
- Elevated heart rate
- Low blood pressure

What Should I Do About Ketoacidosis?

If you are symptomatic:

Ketoacidosis is extremely dangerous and is treated in the hospital. If you have any of the above symptoms, you need to *immediately* call your doctor or go to the nearest emergency room (or both). The bottom line is, if you think something is wrong, it likely is when it comes to ketones.

If you are not yet symptomatic (or not sure):

Check for ketones. If your blood glucose levels are above 240 mg/dL, check for ketones with urine test strips. If you are sick (for example, with a cold or flu or are vomiting for any reason), check for ketones every 4 to 6 hours. If you feel slightly "funky" in any of the ways listed above, go ahead and check.

Have a "game plan" for the future. Everyone should discuss a "game plan" for elevated ketone levels. Some doctors will err on the side of caution and want you to call for "moderate" levels on one test or elevated blood glucose levels that don't seem to be coming down. Others will give you ideas of things to try (such as injections of rapid-acting insulin) after one "moderate" result to bring it down yourself. This strategy should be agreed upon and adhered to strictly.

Call the doctor. If you don't yet have your "game plan" in place for handling ketones, call your doctor immediately if you have high levels of ketones as indicated by a urine test strip (whether or not this is accompanied by high blood glucose levels). You should be extra vigilant if you have vomited and test high. If you test "moderate" two times, call your doctor, unless you have been told otherwise.

How Can I Reduce My Risk of Ketoacidosis?

The following tips will further reduce the likelihood of developing ketoacidosis:

- Test blood glucose very frequently when you are sick: every 2 to 4 hours if you are vomiting, have diarrhea, have a flu or a fever for any reason, every 4 to 6 hours if you have a sore throat or a cold.

- If you have diarrhea, call your doctor if it lasts more than 4 hours. Replace lost fluids by drinking lots of sugar-free, caffeine-free beverages.

- If you are vomiting, call your doctor if it lasts more than 4 hours or if you cannot hold down food or liquid for more than 4 hours.

- Do not exercise on a day when blood glucose has been over 240 mg/dL or if you have had a positive ketone test in the past 24 hours.

Hyperosmolar Hyperglycemic Nonketotic Syndrome (HHNS)

Unlike hypoglycemia or diabetic ketoacidosis, hyperosmolar hyperglycemic nonketotic syndrome (HHNS) is not so acute that it develops within hours, rather it can take days or even weeks to develop. Many people with diabetes have never heard of HHNS. It usually occurs in older people with type 2 diabetes, although it can happen in people with type 1.

HHNS is incredibly dangerous, with a mortality rate of up to 50% in people who develop it. However, since it takes so long to develop, there are plenty of chances to catch it before it gets to this point. The main problem in HHNS is severe dehydration, which results from a repeated cycle of rising blood glucose, excessive urination that further dehydrates, which causes the blood sugar to increase even more. The blood glucose becomes so high—always over 600 mg/dL, but can go as high as 2000 mg/dL—that the blood is actually much more viscous (thicker) from the glucose. Testing for ketones on home test strips will be negative.

What Does HHNS Feel Like and Why Is It Dangerous?

In the early stages of HHNS, the person may feel thirsty, even though they are urinating frequently. As the blood glucose continues to rise, the following symptoms may occur:

- Lethargy or sleepiness
- Nausea, vomiting, or stomach cramps
- Vision becomes blurry or unclear
- There may be a high fever, but no sweating
- The person may be confused or even hallucinate
- There may be weakness on one side of the body

As the process continues, the person may actually become less thirsty and urinate less, and the urine will be very dark in color.

What Should I Do About HHNS?

The following measures can prevent HHNS from becoming life-threatening:

- Continue taking all oral medications and/or insulin
- Test blood glucose frequently, every 2 to 4 hours
- Increase intake of sugar-free, caffeine-free fluids, such as water or diet soda
- Call the doctor if:
  - You have 2 blood glucose readings of 240 mg/dL in a row
  - You have persistent vomiting or diarrhea
  - You are unable to tolerate fluids by mouth for some reason

How Is HHNS Treated?

If blood sugar cannot be brought down or symptoms do not go away at home, HHNS will be treated in the hospital by:

- Rehydrating the person, usually by a combination of IV and oral fluids
- Bringing blood glucose down with insulin and careful monitoring
- Investigating and addressing the cause (treating an infection, for instance)

Long-term Complications

I have tons of complications, despite my bionic efforts to maintain tight control of my blood glucose with my insulin pump and continuous glucose monitoring system (CGMS). No one knows exactly why this is. Maybe it is because there was really no reasonable treatment when I was diagnosed in the early 1970s. However, I know many people diagnosed in the "old days" who have no complications or very few, so this doesn't completely explain things.

However, although I am not comfortable saying that all people with diabetes can *prevent* long-term complications with treatments available today, I will say that they can reduce your risk of these problems by working to maintain control of their blood glucose. It is important to grab control where we can and do what we can for our health, and controlling our blood glucose is an important part of that equation.

At the same time, be vigilant by maintaining scheduled appointments for lab tests and doctor visits to monitor for complications long before you ever experience symptoms. Get to the doctor if you have any concerns. Take action and fight for your health. If you do end up with one of these complications, know that it is not your fault. You can live with these complications and manage them in different ways.

Eye Problems

Diabetes can cause wear and tear on almost every part of our bodies, including damaging the tiny capillaries in the back of our eyes. Although diabetes-related eye problems are common, especially among people with type 1 diabetes, they can often be treated to stop them from getting worse. I know about this from firsthand experience—given what I have been through, the bad news is that I should be blind. The good news is that I'm not.

Diabetic Retinopathy

Diabetic retinopathy is a particularly sensitive subject for me. See, the experts tell us that if we manage to get to 25 years postdiagnosis free of eye problems, then we have won the "golden ticket"—the rest of our lives free of even the worry of developing diabetic retinopathy. In that magical 25th year, my retinologist proclaimed that my retinas were not in danger, saying something to the effect of, "your eyes look so great, it's hard to even tell that you have diabetes." I was ecstatic that there was at least one diabetes-related concern that I could cross off my list forever.

As it turned out, "forever" didn't last very long. Two years later, aggressive proliferative retinopathy came out of nowhere to compromise the vision in my right eye (again defying conventional wisdom that says that retinopathy occurs bilaterally—in both eyes). I first had photocoagulation (often referred to simply as "laser"). I eventually opted for eye surgery after a few years and no more room in my eye for laser, which restored my vision, but shook me up from the sheer strangeness of the experience.

As a side note, I want to tell you that even pretty traumatic situations are easier to endure if you can surround yourself with love and even a couple of laughs to soften the memory of the moment. In the afternoon following my surgery (a vitrectomy), I was sitting at my kitchen table with my patched (and stitched) eye, waiting for the nerve block to wear off so that I could feel the half of my head that had been numb for the past several hours. My brother stopped by the house to see how I was doing. He approached me and grabbed my arms, proclaiming very loudly, "LYNN? IT'S YOUR BROTHER . . . JOHN," as if my eye patch had stolen my ability to hear. I laughed so hard I feared that I might blow another vessel in my retina. The ability to laugh, to find humor, let me know that it was going to be okay. Being able to rely on my brothers for humor in tough situations has proven invaluable in getting through these moments.

The most common form of diabetic retinopathy is "nonproliferative" retinopathy. In this form, the capillaries in the retina become blocked and begin to swell, like fluid-filled balloons. "Proliferative" retinopathy occurs after nonproliferative retinopathy has progressed and the capillaries close off because they are too damaged. To compensate for the loss of these blood vessels, new ones grow in their place. These new capillaries are weak and often leak blood. This can cause vision loss as the blood clouds the vitreous gel. Scar tissue can also form and distort the retina, causing retinal detachment.

What Does Diabetic Retinopathy Feel Like and How Can It Affect My Life? Part of the challenge in keeping diabetic retinopathy under control is that it doesn't really cause too many symptoms in most people until it has already caused significant damage, which is why it is crucial to get your eyes checked regularly.

The symptoms of diabetic retinopathy can include pain in the eye or vision disturbances, such as: blurriness, difficulty reading, seeing floaters, or the sense that there is something blocking your field of vision (partially or totally).

What Can Be Done for Diabetic Retinopathy?
Monitor your eyes. Everyone with type 2 diabetes should undergo a comprehensive eye exam—including dilation—immediately upon diagnosis, and people with type 1 diabetes should get their eyes checked

within 5 years following diagnosis. This should be repeated every year for everyone with diabetes, although some experts say that if you have two or three normal exams, you can have your dilated exam every 2 years instead of every year. (Personally, however, I wouldn't risk waiting that long between exams.)

Photocoagulation. Photocoagulation (often referred to simply as "laser") is the procedure of cauterizing the tiny blood vessels on your retina to stop them from leaking using a laser. In "scatter" or "panretinal" photocoagulation, the doctor uses the laser to make hundreds of tiny burns on your retina—yes, this is almost as "fun" as it sounds. This approach works in the early stages of retinopathy. Focal photocoagulation is used to seal the blood vessels in the macula. If the retinopathy has progressed too far (the retina is already detached or too much blood has leaked into the eye), photocoagulation will not work.

I have to say here that my first experience with photocoagulation was traumatic. I was unprepared for what was going to happen and left feeling scared and shaken—this is another example of how important the right doctor is, as a little more advance warning could have worked wonders. I changed doctors and my next sessions went much more smoothly. Unfortunately, I had a pretty aggressive case of proliferative retinopathy that the laser treatment couldn't keep up with, leading to hemorrhages. I can only describe the result of these hemorrhages, blood that has leaked into the vitreous of my eye, as similar to looking through a lava lamp until the blood was reabsorbed. Eventually, my eye could no longer absorb the blood and I was legally blind in my right eye, and vitrectomy became the best option for restoring my sight.

Vitrectomy. Vitrectomy is what I had, and is the next step if photocoagulation has failed to control the retinopathy. In this procedure, the surgeon makes a tiny incision in the eye and suctions out the vitreous gel, which will clear out all of the blood that has leaked into the vitreous. At this point, he has access to the retina (by inserting surgical instruments into tiny incisions) and may try to reattach the retina, patch holes in the retina or macula or remove scar tissue from the retina. After all repairs are done, the vitreous gel in the eye is replaced with saline solution or silicone oil (eventually the body will replace this material with vitreous).

Vitrectomy totally restored my sight. I went from blind in that eye to not blind in one day! Now that you know the happy ending, I will tell you that the vitrectomy procedure was rather bizarre, to say the least.

Much of my surgery was done under local anesthesia and I was aware of what was happening—the laser cauterization of the retina brought to mind a wood burning kit that my brothers had as kids (so went my thoughts under heavy doses of drugs). Fortunately, the least pleasant part (the stitching of the eyeball) is now done only rarely, as the incisions in the eye are now much smaller and the sclera can heal itself.

Cataracts

A cataract is clouding of the lens of the eye. Although conventional wisdom tells us that if we live long enough, we will all develop cataracts, those of us with diabetes are much more likely to develop them at an earlier age. Vitrectomies also greatly increase the risk of developing a cataract at a younger age.

What Do Cataracts Feel Like and How Can They Affect My Life? At first, you will not be able to see a cataract and may not even be aware that one is developing, as your eyes work to compensate for any vision loss. Eventually, you may notice a cloudiness or blurring of your vision. Other symptoms of cataracts include: double vision (usually only in one eye), distorted colors, halos around lights, sensitivity to light, reduced night vision. You may not notice anything in particular, but find yourself wishing that there was more light to read by or not be satisfied with vision improvement from glasses or contacts that worked just fine a couple of months ago.

What Can Be Done for Cataracts? Unfortunately, we currently have no drugs or supplements to treat cataracts and glasses and contact lenses really won't help you see better as the cataract progresses (although you may be able to compensate for a while with brighter lights or higher magnification). Pretty much the only way to treat a cataract is to remove the cloudy lens, replacing it with an artificial lens. This is a pretty routine operation that usually has excellent outcomes. An added bonus for some people is that a corrective lens can be implanted to compensate for any vision problems, resulting in better vision than was had before the cataract.

Glaucoma

The risk of glaucoma for people with diabetes may be almost twice as high as for the general population, although other experts say the link is weaker than that. Glaucoma is increased pressure in the eye, caused by a slow drainage of the fluid in the eye. This pressure "squeezes" or constricts the blood vessels in the eye, which can damage the optic nerve or retina and lead to vision loss.

What Does Glaucoma Feel Like and How Can It Affect My Life? The most common type of glaucoma is open-angle glaucoma. Open angle glaucoma doesn't usually have any symptoms until significant damage has been done. The first noticeable symptom is usually loss of peripheral vision. Neovascular glaucoma can be caused by diabetic retinopathy, occurring when new blood vessels grow on the iris. It can cause severe vision loss.

What Can Be Done for Glaucoma?

Eye drops. For most people, glaucoma can be successfully treated with eye drops that work to reduce the pressure in the eye. Some of these work by improving fluid drainage, and others work to reduce the amount of aqueous fluid made by the eye.

Laser treatment. There are several types of laser surgery for glaucoma: laser trabeculoplasty improves outflow of aqueous fluid by making 50 to 100 tiny burns in the structure that allows the fluid to drain out of the eye; peripheral iridotomy creates a tiny hole in the iris, to allow the pressure in front and in back of the iris to equalize; laser cyclophotocoagulation destroys small parts of the structure that makes aqueous fluid so that less is made. Retinal photocoagulation to reduce abnormal blood vessels on the retina and iris may be successful in treating neovascular glaucoma.

Surgery. The simplest form of surgery is called trabeculectomy or a sclerostomy, where the surgeon makes a small opening in the sclera to create a new drainage path. Drainage implants can be surgically placed to help regulate pressure within the eye.

Nerve Problems

Up to 70% of all people with diabetes will experience a neuropathy, or nerve disorder. The most common neuropathies linked to diabetes are peripheral neuropathy and autonomic neuropathy, which are discussed in more detail below. Although neuropathies are the most common complication of diabetes, no one is entirely sure of their exact cause. It is widely thought that there is a combination of factors at work, including damage to the tiny blood vessels that bring oxygen and nutrients to the nerves, as well as chronic inflammation and metabolic factors that may cause destruction of the axons (nerve fibers).

The body is operated by a vast system of nerves, and virtually all of them are vulnerable to damage. Therefore, the list of possible ways these nerves can malfunction is also quite long. Bottom line: if you have pain, tingling or weakness in any area of your body, see your doctor to determine the cause, get as much relief as you can, and prevent further damage or other health consequences that might be linked to a particular neuropathy.

Peripheral Neuropathy

Peripheral neuropathy is a problem with the nerves that transmit signals to the brain and spinal cord from other parts of the body.

What Does Peripheral Neuropathy Feel Like and How Can It Affect My Life?
Peripheral neuropathy feels different, depending on the person and depending on how long it has been happening, meaning how much damage has already occurred. Peripheral neuropathy (also known as sensorimotor neuropathy) typically affects the toes, feet and legs, although the hands and arms can also be affected. At the beginning, it may feel like tingling or "pins and needles" in the feet, like when your foot "falls asleep." It may also feel like you have socks on when you don't. It might feel like your feet are very cold or hot, even though they do not feel different to the touch. These sensations may be worse at night or when your feet are being touched.

Other people may skip the tingling phase and feel pain in their feet. This may feel like burning or it may feel like "walking on rocks."

Eventually, if damage progresses, all feeling is lost in the feet. They are completely numb with no feeling in them even when you are walking or if you hurt your foot. You are unable to feel difference in temperatures, even when there is extreme hot or cold. This numbness may make it difficult to walk smoothly, and make the muscles in your legs and feet feel weak.

What Can Be Done About Peripheral Neuropathy? To reduce the likelihood of developing peripheral neuropathy, keeping blood glucose in the target range might help. However, this is one of the first long-term complications to show up, and it is possible that you will not be able to completely prevent it because of high blood glucose before diagnosis or other factors that make you susceptible to nerve damage.

There is really no way to cure peripheral neuropathies. Some people find that gaining tighter control over their blood glucose can eventually lessen the sensations, but often feel more intense symptoms at the beginning of tight glucose control. However, there are things to be done to dull the pain or ease discomfort of peripheral neuropathy.

See a neurologist. You may want to be evaluated and treated by a neurologist for your peripheral neuropathy (or at least get a referral, especially if your diabetes is being treated by a general practitioner), as these specialists can evaluate how extensive the damage is and have experience with the different medications and approaches to lessening discomfort.

Oral medications. There are several oral meds that your doctor can try to help with painful peripheral neuropathy, including tricyclic antidepressants, newer forms of antidepressants, opiates or anticonvulsants. This may require some trial and error, as different classes of meds are more effective in some people than others and all of these drugs have side effects. It should be noted that most people do not get much relief from the nonsteroidal anti-inflammatory drugs (NSAIDs), such as paracetamol (Tylenol) or ibuprofen (Motrin), so these are generally not recommended for neuropathies.

Topical treatments. Most of the best creams to treat peripheral neuropathy contain capsaicin, the same ingredient found in hot peppers. Some people also find relief from patches that contain lidocaine or sprays that contain nitrate.

Alternative medicine. Some people find relief from complementary and alternative medicine approaches, like acupuncture, transcutaneous electrical nerve stimulation (TENS), biofeedback, and certain supplements (alpha-lipoic acid or evening primrose oil). Discuss any of these that you may be interested in with your doctor. Read the blogs on this topic as well—I have learned great tips on the Internet, such as standing on a cool tile floor in the middle of the night to dull the sensations long enough to get back to sleep.

Autonomic Neuropathy

Unless one is a physician, researcher, or physical therapist, the average person does not spend a great deal of time actually thinking about why the different parts of the body and organ systems work until they stop working. The process becomes a little more interesting as we strive to restore function where possible.

The variety of autonomic neuropathy symptoms really points to how much of what goes on inside of us is controlled by the autonomic nerves, as many of our bodily functions are negatively impacted when the autonomic nerves are damaged, including digestion, urination, vision, sexual response, respiration, and cardiac function (among others). Autonomic neuropathy also can reduce or eliminate the signals that hypoglycemia is occurring, such as feeling shaky or light-headed, making a person unaware that this is happening until they lose consciousness (called hypoglycemic unawareness).

What Does Autonomic Neuropathy Feel Like and How Can It Affect My Life?
Because the autonomic nervous system controls pretty much all of our organs, the symptoms vary by organ system that is damaged. Here are some of the possible effects of autonomic neuropathy on different organs:

Heart or vascular system. These symptoms can include dizziness, feeling lightheaded, or fainting upon standing quickly. This is caused by a delay of the heart increasing output and a drop in blood pressure. People can also experience a rapid resting heartbeat or be unable to exercise because the heart does not respond to activity levels and the heart rate stays "stuck" in one place. People can also experience heart attacks without typical warning signs.

Digestive system. When the nerves of the intestines are involved, "diabetic diarrhea" can occur, with people having many bowel movements a day. Fecal incontinence (losing control of the bowels) can also happen. The other side of the spectrum is constipation, which is one of the most common autonomic neuropathies. Gastroparesis (covered separately below) is a form of autonomic neuropathy, which has symptoms such as heartburn, bloated feeling after eating, nausea and vomiting.

Eye and optic nerve. The autonomic nerves in the eye that can be affected are those of the pupil, which controls how much light comes into the eye. Neuropathy of these nerves leads to difficulty adjusting to differences in lighting, such going into a bright place at night or turning off a light, as the pupil is very slow to react. This can also cause problems seeing in the dark, particularly while driving at night.

Urinary tract. These symptoms take the form of difficulties voiding urine from the body, including incontinence or losing control of your bladder, loss of sensation or needing to urinate even when bladder is full, or feeling the need to urinate when there is no urine in the bladder. These problems often result in residual urine staying in the bladder, which leads to bladder infections. Fortunately, there are medications to treat the different ways that the bladder is "malfunctioning," which work in various ways like increasing bladder contraction or decreasing urine output.

Sexual functioning. Both men and women can be affected by neuropathies of the sexual organs (covered in more detail below). Male problems include maintaining an erection or ejaculating. Women often have difficulty with vaginal dryness or achieving orgasm.

Perspiration. Sweating symptoms can include excessive sweating or not sweating at all. Often the feet do not sweat at all, leading to heavy perspiration in other places as the body tries to compensate. Some people sweat excessively after eating spicy food or cheese. This can often be treated with a scopolamine patch or, more recently, Botox has successfully been used to treat excessive perspiration.

What Can Be Done About Autonomic Neuropathy? Fortunately, many of the symptoms of the various autonomic neuropathies can be managed to some extent. However, the disappointing news is that none of them can be actually "cured"—all of the available approaches target reducing the symptoms to lessen negative impact on your life.

One of my favorite stories about living with diabetes with confidence is related to my own experience in trying to grapple with my autonomic neuropathies. I have gastroparesis, which comes and goes, ranging from irritating to debilitating. I also have a relatively rare form of cardiac neuropathy, which does a great job of reminding me that it's not all about blood sugar control. It is the unpredictable nature of these things that may be the most draining.

During one appointment with my wonderful endocrinologist, he and I were working our way down the list of my current "challenges," including my autonomic neuropathies. My endo was listening intently to my description of symptoms around my gastroparesis, while taking notes and throwing out the occasional tip, such as "we need to work on ways to avoid vomiting as much as possible, as you don't want to blow out those vulnerable blood vessels in your retina." He then proceeded to continue working his way down the list of other possibilities of things that might come up in my future, asking matter-of-factly, "Have you lost control of your bowels yet?" I replied, "Thankfully, no. However, could you please not add the word 'YET' to the end of that question!?"

Gastroparesis

Although gastroparesis falls under the category of autonomic neuropathy, I felt it deserved its own special entry by me, because it is one of the complications that I have grappled with. Put simply, gastroparesis is delayed emptying of the stomach. This happens because the nerve which usually causes the stomach to contract (the vagus nerve) to move the food along into the small intestine is damaged, and the food just sits in the stomach.

What Does Gastroparesis Feel Like and How Can It Affect My Life?

Like many of these complications, a mere listing of the symptoms of gastroparesis does not do justice to the discomfort and pain it actually causes the individual. However, for the sake of completeness, the symptoms of gastroparesis can be any of the following, alone or in combination: appetite loss, vomiting and nausea, heartburn and/or gastroesophageal reflux, feelings of fullness or bloating (even after just a couple bites of food), abdominal pain or spasms, and weight loss.

What Can Be Done About Gastroparesis?

I'll be honest here. There is no wonderful treatment for gastroparesis—at least I have not found it. At least it seems to come and go, but it is different for everyone. My best advice is to immediately stop eating big meals and fiber when you have symptoms and move to liquids (my favorite is tomato soup) if it lasts too long. I do everything I can to avoid vomiting because: 1) seeing undigested food come up is gross and gives me an unattractive deep bass voice for days, and 2) vomiting completely wipes me out—if I vomit, I am in bed for the rest of the day. Strangely, some other people that I know feel like their stomach is "reset" after vomiting and their gastroparesis symptoms are greatly diminished. Here are some details on what might work for you:

Make some dietary changes (permanent or temporary). Avoid high-fat and high-fiber foods. Eat lots of tiny meals instead of a few large ones. Eat (drink) liquid or pureed foods.

Medications. Taken before meals and at bedtime, metoclopramide (Reglan) speeds stomach emptying by stimulating the stomach muscles to contract. For many people, it also reduces nausea and vomiting. However, metoclopramide comes with side effects, which can include sleepiness, depression, or anxiety. (Personally this drug did nothing to improve my condition and the side effects were not worth the suffering with no noticeable benefit.) Some doctors use the "side effects" of intense stomach contractions that come with the antibiotic erythromycin to help people with gastroparesis, as this drug improves stomach emptying and moves food through the stomach when taken on a regular schedule.

Closely watch blood glucose levels. Increased monitoring of blood glucose may be needed when you have gastroparesis, as food absorption is not usual. Depending on how much you are (or are not) digesting, you may become hypoglycemic after a meal if you take your normal amount of insulin—treating this hypoglycemia might involve drinking liquids or eating something like honey that is very quickly absorbed. You and your doctor may have to strategize and adapt your treatment during this time.

Be patient. Although easier said than done, you may just have to wait out your gastroparesis. For most of us, gastroparesis comes and goes, especially the most severe problems. I have had gastroparesis for almost 30 years and have only had two instances, lasting about a week each time, during which I had to consume an entirely liquid diet. I usually get enough warning in the form of a bloated feeling immediately after eating or hypoglycemia that tells me I should cut way back on volume for a few days—by heeding what my body is telling me, I believe I have been able to avert more severe problems.

Foot Problems

Perhaps more than any other complication from diabetes, really serious foot problems are a bit more preventable, as they usually start out as pretty minor foot problems that can be caught and treated before they lead to more extreme medical situations.

What Do Foot Problems Feel Like and How Can They Affect My Life?

Foot problems don't really "feel" like anything once the nerves are damaged and sensation is lost, which is the root of the whole problem. (Prior to losing sensation, peripheral neuropathy can be extremely painful as described above.) Eventually peripheral neuropathy leads to loss of sensation in the foot, so that people do not feel when there has been an injury to the foot. Injuries to the foot, such as ulcers, are common because there is poor circulation in the foot (making the skin more fragile, drier, and prone to calluses), and there are changes to the shape of the foot due to nerve damage. All of this is made worse by the fact that diabetes makes us more prone to infections because of poor circulation and high glucose in the blood (which microorganisms thrive on).

What Can Be Done About Foot Problems?

The first tactic is to prevent any sort of injury to the foot. Some of the tips around this are:

- *Seek and destroy.* Thoroughly examine your feet nightly. If you have a hard time seeing the bottom of your feet, invest in a handheld mirror or see if you can persuade a family member to take over this duty. See a doctor immediately if you find a sore or an area of redness on your foot. Ensure that your doctor checks your feet at least twice yearly. Make a habit of taking off your shoes before the doctor enters the room at your appointments—it's a reminder to both of you.

- *Use a monofilament to test the sensation in your feet.* A monofilament is a thin piece of plastic string that is a precise size, so that it does not bend until 10 grams of pressure is applied. If you (or your doctor) is able to press it against the bottom of your foot and bend it without you feeling it, this indicates that you have lost enough protective sensation in your feet to put you at significantly increased risk of ulcers from minor injuries that go undetected. It is actually fairly difficult to find one that is accurate. Ask your doctor about this, as he might be able to give you one or tell you where to get your own monofilament.

- *Consult a shoe expert.* Consider seeing a pedorthist (www.pedorthics.org), a person who is certified to basically make sure that shoes fit, especially for people with feet that are vulnerable for some reason.

- *"Ugly" shoes.* They don't have to be super-ugly, but shoes need to fit well, not too loose and not too tight from the moment you buy them. They need to be well-cushioned. They should not have pointy toes or high heels. Although these criteria seem to be excluding many of the really cute shoes out there, with some persistence, you can find some shoes that have some redeeming fashion features. The same shoes should not be worn 2 days in a row.

  I have to say here that the above paragraph is really only relevant if you have numb areas on your feet or circulatory problems of the lower extremities. It is one of my biggest pet peeves that all of the foot care information for people with diabetes assumes that none of us can feel our feet. I can, so I wear heels and occasionally even shoes with pointy toes.

- *Stop smoking.* Although I do not have the space to devote to the importance of this or how to do it, this cannot go unmentioned. For so many reasons, if you have diabetes, you need to stop smoking. There, I said it (and in a much nicer way than many authors, who simply say "keep smoking if you want an amputation").

- *Deal with calluses.* Use a pumice stone and keep feet moisturized.

Although I would like to believe that everyone will do everything on the above list, I know that most people (including myself) won't. Because "all or nothing" strategies rarely work in real life, you must use logic and apply it consistently. For instance, I love the beach; furthermore, I love to walk barefoot on the beach. Although this is a huge no-no according to every brochure for patients with diabetes, I have avoided problems by thoroughly examining my feet after each time I go barefoot. Live your life, but do what you have to in order to be safe.

If you do find a sore, take it very seriously. See your doctor immediately and stay off of your feet as much as possible until it is healed. Follow self-care instructions to the letter. Almost all serious foot problems started with a minor injury that could have been treated if caught early and addressed.

Complications Involving the Heart and Blood Vessels

High blood pressure, high serum cholesterol, high triglycerides, increased risk of heart attack, higher incidence of stroke, peripheral artery disease—all of these things are much more common and much more dangerous in people with diabetes. As we know, all of these things are related and are very difficult to discuss in isolation, especially in regard to reducing the occurrence of these problems.

Therefore, I am going to get that little talk out of the way early and tell you what you already know in terms of things we can all do to reduce our risk of these things. Again, we all know these prevention tips, as they are not specific to people with diabetes, but they apply to everyone:

- Eat better—reduce fat and sodium
- Maintain a healthy weight
- Exercise
- Quit smoking
- Use alcohol in moderation

There. I'm going to assume there is nothing on that list that comes as a surprise. In addition to these things, you and your doctor may decide to take the following preventive measures, depending on your risk factors, as well as his or her particular approach to reducing risk of these complications:

- Statins
- Low-dose aspirin therapy
- Angiotensin-converting enzyme (ACE) inhibitors

I will move along to briefly discuss the particulars of each complication of the heart and blood vessels.

Increased Risk of Heart Attack

People with diabetes are more likely than other people to have a heart attack for many reasons. In fact, even when people with diabetes did the things to reduce their risk of heart disease—stop smoking and lower cholesterol and blood pressure—they still have the same risk of having a heart attack as people without diabetes who have already had a heart attack (although much better than it would be had they not taken those measures).[4]

What Does a Heart Attack Feel Like? What Are the Warning Signs of a Heart Attack?

- **Chest discomfort.** Most heart attacks involve discomfort in the center of the chest that lasts more than a few minutes or that goes away and comes back. It can feel like uncomfortable pressure, squeezing, fullness or pain.
- **Discomfort in other areas of the upper body.** Symptoms can include pain or discomfort in one or both arms, the back, neck, jaw, or stomach.
- **Shortness of breath** with or without chest discomfort.
- **Other signs** may include breaking out in a cold sweat, nausea or lightheadedness.

As with men, women's most common heart attack symptom is chest pain or discomfort. But women are somewhat more likely than men to experience some of the other common symptoms, particularly shortness of breath, nausea /vomiting, and back or jaw pain.

What Should I Do if I Think I Am Having a Heart Attack?

Call 911 immediately. Don't wait to "see what happens" if you think you are having a heart attack. Minutes count here. In most cases, it's better to call 911 than have someone drive you to the hospital, because paramedics can start treatment and evaluation on the way.

Take aspirin. After calling 911, chew (don't swallow) one adult-strength aspirin (325 mg) or two to four baby aspirin (81 mg each), unless you have an allergy or other reason not to take aspirin.

Make a plan with your doctor. If you have risk factors for a heart attack, you should discuss an "emergency plan" with your doctor—he may want you to take additional steps, like take a beta-blocker right after calling 911.

Increased Risk of Stroke

A stroke can happen for one of two reasons—the blood flow to part of the brain is blocked by a blood clot (called ischemic stroke) or there is bleeding in the brain from a ruptured blood vessel (called hemorrhagic stroke). People with diabetes are at extra risk from strokes. A friend of mine with type 1 diabetes has had three strokes in recent years, despite taking the best possible care of herself with the tools we had on hand at the time.

What Does a Stroke Feel Like? What Are the Warning Signs of a Stroke?

Warning signs of a stroke come on suddenly. They can include any of the following:

- Severe headache
- Weakness or numbness on one side of your body
- Trouble talking so that people can understand you
- Trouble understanding others or general confusion
- Balance issues or trouble walking
- Trouble seeing out of one or both eyes or double vision

If you have any of these symptoms that come on suddenly, then disappear, you may have had a TIA (transient ischemic attack). TIAs (also referred to by some as "mini strokes") are caused by a temporary block-age of blood flow to a certain area of the brain. They differ from true strokes because they only last for a short time and do not leave perma-nent damage. See a doctor if you think you have experienced a TIA.

What Should I Do if I Think I Am Having a Stroke?

Call 911 immediately. Minutes matter in treating a stroke, in terms of pre-venting potential permanent damage (or death).

Teach relatives and others to recognize signs of a stroke. There is a simple "3-step test" that anyone can use to diagnose probable strokes:

- Ask the person to "smile" or "show me your teeth." Look for signs that one side of the face is weak—the smile will be lopsided.

- Ask the person to close their eyes and raise their arms. Look to see if one side is weaker than the other—both arms will not be raised to the same height or one will drift to the side.

- Look for signs of slurred speech or problems by asking someone to repeat a simple phrase. Try something easy like "don't cry over spilled milk" or "it looks like rain today."

Do not *take aspirin.*

Peripheral Artery Disease (PAD)

While about one-third of people with diabetes have PAD, half of these people do not realize that they have it. PAD is a condition where there is insufficient blood flow to your feet and legs because the blood vessels in the legs are narrowed or blocked by fatty deposits.

What Does PAD Feel Like and How Can It Affect My Life? Many people with PAD don't have any symptoms, or their symptoms are so mild that they don't think they are anything to worry about. Some people have one or more of the following symptoms:

- Leg pain, feelings of heaviness, or cramping of the legs when walking, exercising, or climbing stairs. These sensations usu-ally go away after a few minutes of rest. This is called "inter-mittent claudation."

- Numbness, tingling, or coldness in the lower legs or feet, which may be more noticeable in one leg as compared to the other.

- Sores or infections on your feet or legs that heal slowly and/or decreased hair growth on the legs and weak toenails.

- The skin on the legs being unusually pale or slightly blue.

What Can Be Done About PAD?

Have it diagnosed. The easiest test is the ankle brachial index, which is simply a test to measure the blood pressure in your lower leg. If it is lower than the blood pressure in your arm, you may have PAD. To figure out which specific blood vessels are blocked, the following tests may be performed: angiogram (X-rays are taken of the legs after dye is injected), Doppler ultrasound or MRI. You may also be asked to walk on a treadmill to determine how severe your symptoms are and what level of exertion brings them on.

Blood-thinning medications. These may be prescribed to try to dissolve the blockage or prevent clots from forming.

Angioplasty. This is done by inserting a small catheter with a balloon into the blocked or narrowed artery, then inflating it to widen the artery and restore blood flow. A stent (small mesh tube) may be placed in the artery to help keep it open.

Bypass grafting. In this procedure, a blood vessel from another part of your body (or an artificial one) is surgically attached to the artery on either side of the blockage, essentially allowing the blood to flow around it.

High Blood Pressure

High blood pressure (hypertension), defined as blood pressure that is higher than 140/90 mm Hg, affects an estimated 60% of people with diabetes.

What Does Hypertension Feel Like and How Can It Affect My Life? In most cases, hypertension feels like . . . nothing. In most cases, there are absolutely *no* symptoms of hypertension. However, in rare cases (or when blood pressure spikes suddenly for some reason) a person can experience headaches, fatigue, dizziness, confusion, ringing in the ears (tinnitus), blurred vision, difficulty breathing, palpitations (irregular or pounding heartbeat), or nosebleeds.

If you are having any of these symptoms, it is crucial to see a doctor right away, as this could mean that a heart attack or stroke could follow.

What Can Be Done About Hypertension? The current target blood pressure for people with diabetes is 130/80 mm Hg. However, this may be revisited in the future, as one study showed an increased risk of stroke, heart attack or death when systolic blood pressure was brought below 130 as opposed to keeping it between 130 and 140.[5]

Medication. ACE inhibitors lower blood pressure by keeping your blood vessels relaxed. ACE inhibitors prevent a hormone called angiotensin from forming in your body and narrowing your blood vessels. ACE inhibitors also help protect your kidneys and reduce your risk of heart attack and stroke. This is a first-line hypertension drug class for people with diabetes, as they have also been shown to reduce the risk of diabetic retinopathy. Many doctors add other drugs to the drug regimen to treat hypertension, such as beta-blockers, calcium channel blockers, or diuretics.

High Cholesterol

For most people with diabetes, the target cholesterol/lipid levels are total serum cholesterol below 200; LDL (bad) cholesterol below 100; HDL (good) cholesterol above 40 in men and above 50 in women; triglycerides below 150. If someone with diabetes has overt cardiovascular disease, the recommendations are to get LDL below 70 mg/dL.

What Does High Cholesterol Feel Like and How Can It Affect My Life? There are no symptoms of high cholesterol. However, high cholesterol means that you are at a greatly increased risk of having a heart attack or stroke.

What Can Be Done About High Cholesterol?
Statins. Many people with diabetes take one of the statins—atorvastatin, fluvastatin, lovastatin, pravastatin, or simvastatin. In

fact, it is recommended by the American Diabetes Association that statins be taken by anyone with diabetes who is over 40 and has other risk factors for cardiovascular disease (such as family history of heart problems, hypertension, smoking, etc.), regardless of cholesterol levels at baseline.[6] There was some attention in the media of statins contributing to risk of developing type 2 diabetes, but this risk is extremely small, and the benefits of taking statins for someone who already has diabetes are well-proven, with some studies showing as much as a 19% to 55% reduction in risk of a heart attack or stroke.[7]

Kidney Problems/Diabetic Nephropathy

Although diabetic retinopathy and kidney problems usually occur together—as the tiny blood vessels on the retinas and in the kidneys are similar in size and structure, and therefore seem to be similarly vulnerable—I have not added kidney issues to my list of complications (although I have diabetic retinopathy). Since I mistakenly thought I was "off the hook" for retinopathy after I passed the 25-year mark, only to be slammed a couple of years later, I am pretty vigilant about keeping my blood pressure under control, which is an important component of protecting our kidneys.

What Do Diabetic Kidney Problems Feel Like and How Can They Affect My Life?

In the beginning stages, kidney problems in people with diabetes do not have any symptoms—in fact, these problems could be developing for 10 years or more before any symptoms show up and up to 15 years before they become so bothersome that they lead someone to a doctor. The symptoms of more advanced diabetic nephropathy include reduced urine output, headache, fatigue, nausea, decreased appetite, overall malaise or feeling sick, swelling of the legs, around the eyes or the entire body (so much that weight gain is noticed). There can also be strange symptoms like itching all over the body or hiccups. People may notice that the urine in the toilet is very foamy or frothy.

What Can Be Done About Diabetic Kidney Problems?

Get tested for microalbuminuria with a 24-hour urine test. This is a test that can find out if your kidneys are in the early stages of kidney disease several years before a dipstick would reveal high levels.

Improve cholesterol levels. Like many other people, those with diabetes are trying to improve their LDL (bad cholesterol)/HDL (good cholesterol) ratio, as well as bring down triglyceride numbers. Diet can help, but many people have found that statins are really needed to get these levels where they should be.

Bring blood pressure down. Avoid salt. Take angiotensin-converting enzyme (ACE) inhibitors and/or angiotensin receptor blockers (ARBs).

Prevent urinary tract infections. Urinary tract infections can damage the kidneys. People with diabetes often have issues with the nerves that monitor bladder capacity, leading to problems with bladder emptying. This results in stagnant urine, which is a perfect environment for a bladder infection.

Avoid certain things. People with kidney dysfunction need to take extra precautions to avoid anything that might put too much strain on their kidneys, such as certain dyes and contrast agents used in diagnostic scans and imaging (make sure the doctors and technicians are aware of your kidney problems); NSAIDs, which include many over-the-counter pain relievers, such as ibuprofen, naproxen, and aspirin, as well as some prescription-strength pain relievers; and COX-2 inhibitors, such as Celebrex.

Dialysis/transplant. If kidney dysfunction progresses, dialysis may be necessary. Dialysis is a process that periodically removes wastes from the blood by passing it through a filter, either using an external machine (hemodialysis) or a system implanted in the person's abdomen (peritoneal dialysis). Some people may go on to have a kidney transplant, which are very successful in the majority (85%–95%) of cases. A special note is that every year around a thousand people in the United States have a combined kidney/pancreas transplant.[8] In many cases, the transplanted pancreas will take over the functioning of the recipient's original destroyed beta cells, in essence "curing" the transplant recipient of diabetes, although this may not be permanent. For those interested in learning more about this, Deb Butterfield chronicles her pancreas transplant in her book, *Showdown with Diabetes*, which also contains information about islet cell transplantation.

Sexual Dysfunction

What Does Diabetes-related Sexual Dysfunction Feel Like and How Can It Affect My Life?

Women with diabetes may experience a range of sexual problems, including vaginal dryness, reduced sensation or exaggerated sensitivity in the vaginal area, difficulty with the movements and positions involved in sex due to pain or muscle spasms, loss of libido (interest in sex), and difficulty having orgasms. Men with diabetes may experience the following sexual problems: reduced sensitivity in the penis, difficulty getting or keeping an erection (erectile dysfunction), difficulty with ejaculation (dry orgasm), loss of libido.

For both sexes, sexual dysfunction can harm or even destroy a relationship, especially if there is not good communication.

What Can Be Done about Diabetes-related Sexual Dysfunction?

Communication with your partner is by far the most important component of the solution to sexual dysfunction, and often the most difficult. Men and women with diabetes are probably already experiencing some degree of embarrassment about the situation, so bringing up the subject of sexual dysfunction may be frightening. It is also crucial to seek help from your doctor even though this may be uncomfortable. Many treatments exist for both female and male sexual dysfunction, but your doctor cannot help you with your sexual concerns unless you mention them.

Medical approaches for men experiencing erectile dysfunction can include medications such as Viagra and Cialis, which work in most men with diabetes. There are also medications that can be injected into the base of the penis to produce an erection and devices that can be surgically inserted into the penis to assist with erections. Women can often get help from vaginal lubricants or vibrators, and some medications, such as Viagra, work to help women with arousal.

Expanding your concept of sex beyond orgasms, to include hugging, kissing and other forms of contact, will keep the intimacy alive.

Depression

Research shows that people with diabetes are twice as likely to become depressed as people without diabetes.[9] There may be physical effects of diabetes on the brain that contributes to depression, but people can also get depressed from the emotional burden of dealing with diabetes or its complications, the constant demands of managing the disease, feelings of guilt or perceived blame from loved ones, or fear of the unknown.

What Does Depression Feel Like and How Can it Affect My Life?

According to the *Diagnostic and Statistical Manual of Mental Disorders, Fourth Edition (DSM-IV)*, the diagnostic manual of the American Psychiatric Association that contains the criteria used by mental health professionals to diagnose people, you are clinically depressed if you have had at least five of the following symptoms, representing a change in function, for at least 2 weeks: sadness, loss of interest in things you previously liked to do, change in appetite, problems sleeping, moving faster or slower than usual (so that people notice), fatigue, feelings of guilt, cognitive problems, or suicidal thoughts. In addition, the symptoms must be severe enough to upset your daily routine, seriously impair your work, or interfere with your relationships and is not just a normal reaction to the death of a loved one.

The Real World

While depressed, you may not have the insight to realize that you are depressed. Be sure a loved one whom you talk with frequently knows the signs of depression and what to do about it.

According to the *DSM-IV*, clinical depression does not have a specific cause like alcohol, drugs, medication side effects, or physical illness. There is a spectrum of depression—people who are on one end may feel sluggish and less enthusiastic about some things. On the other end of the spectrum, depression can be debilitating and untreated depression can lead to suicide.

What Can Be Done About Depression?

Depression is particularly evil, as it can mercilessly target and erode the very resolve that you need in order to fight it, and certainly can have a negative impact on how much attention we can give to managing our diabetes. The pain can be worse than physical pain, and be just as immobilizing. Remember, depression is not your fault. It is not a sign of weakness, and nothing to be embarrassed about, however, you must fight it if it comes. You have no choice.

Whether you meet all of the necessary criteria for depression or not—it doesn't matter in terms of what you need to do next. If you feel very sad or have no interest in things around you, you absolutely need to seek help as soon as possible. Leave the diagnosis and treatment to a professional. Although any physician can prescribe antidepressant medications, I *highly* recommend that you see a psychiatrist for any suspected depression.

The treatment of depression requires careful monitoring and individualized treatment plans. A psychiatrist has experience with all forms of depression and has observed the effects of different medications firsthand. She will be able to tell you what to expect and ask the right questions to allow her to adjust your dose over time to ensure the best response possible. There are many medications that are effective against depression, but often it is a matter of trial and error before exactly the right combination and dosages are determined. Research has shown that combining treatment with medications with psychotherapy (talk therapy) is the most effective treatment of depression. Depending on what is available in your area and what you are comfortable with, this can be in the form of individual, one-on-one sessions or in a group setting. Ideally, you could find a psychologist or counselor who had experience working with people with diabetes.

I'll say it again—it is important that you get help to feel better. All of us living with diabetes have more than enough to deal with and depression can affect the course of our illness, because it can impact how well or poorly we take care of ourselves.

Pregnancy Risks

Pregnancy and diabetes can be a rough combination, as hormones in pregnancy can wreak havoc with blood glucose, which in turn can cause problems for an unborn baby. This subject is complex and way beyond the scope of this book. However, there is an excellent book that covers the information in a refreshing and informative way. *Balancing Pregnancy with Pre-Existing Diabetes* by Cheryl Alkon is written by a woman with type 1 diabetes who has been through it herself. It is a comprehensive guide to those things that might worry a mom-to-be with diabetes, including everything from preconception and planning to the postpartum period, with special information about fertility treatments and miscarriage. One of my favorite sections is called "Explaining Yourself and the *Steel Magnolias* Mindset," where she specifically addresses the judgment and concern coming from friends and family and gives tips on how to "deal with the commentary." If you are a woman with diabetes (or in a relationship with one) who is planning on having a baby (or already pregnant), this book is a must-read.

How to Talk to Your Doctor About Your Symptoms

When we visit our doctor often the most helpful information he or she has is the details that we can give about the symptom and our experiences, especially in the symptoms that we feel (like pain or fatigue) more than those that can be measured objectively (like vision or high blood pressure). There are treatments that can help most symptoms, but the doctor must be able to determine the most likely cause and how much it is affecting your life before knowing what course to try and how aggressive to be in a symptom management approach.

Here are some questions the doctor might ask about a symptom—let's use peripheral neuropathy as our example:

How would you describe your symptom? Here, you can get descriptive and give answers like "it feels like a million ants are biting me" or "it feels like I am wearing socks made of AstroTurf." Answer with as much detail as you can, avoiding simple, vague answers like "it feels kinda weird."

How long does the sensation typically last? The doctor may be trying to determine if the tingling or burning is directly because of high blood glucose, indicating that damage is occurring, or that blood glucose is better controlled and healing is beginning, which can be uncomfortable.

What is the correlation with your blood glucose levels? Your doctor will want to know what is happening here—is the neuropathy worse when your blood glucose is low? When it is high? Is there no correlation at all?

When is it the worst? Do you feel worse when you first wake up or does the tingling and burning seem to worsen as the day wears on? Does it get worse an hour after you have taken a certain medication?

How intense is the sensation? See if you can rate your burning or tingling feeling on a scale of 1 to 10—with "1" being a very slight tickle and "10" being the feeling of excruciating raw pain (or worse).

Does the symptom affect your daily activities? Have the neuropathy sensations kept you home from work? Have you not kept up with your usual chores around the house because of the fatigue? Have there been any times that you were supposed to spend time with friends and family that you canceled or not engaged in your favorite hobbies because of the pain? Has your pain affected your sex life?

Have you noticed that anything makes it feel better or worse? Think hard about this one. Does the burning or tingling get more intense when you go to bed? Is the sensation worsened by stress?

How effective are your neuropathy medications or home remedies? Talk about all medications and remedies that you have tried for your neuropathy, including over-the-counter drugs and any illegal drugs you may have tried (it is important to tell all of these things to the doctor, even if you are pretty sure he will not think it was a good idea to use these things). Rate their effects on a scale of 1 to 10—"1" being that you detected no effect at all and "10" meaning that the sensation quickly and completely disappeared. Also mention any other things you may have tried, including acupuncture, massage, biofeedback, or other complementary and alternative methods.

Again, the above example used peripheral neuropathy for the sake of illustrating the kinds of details doctors want to know about symptoms. Think about any symptom or complication (hypoglycemia, gastroparesis, sexual dysfunction) that you might want to discuss with your doctor with a similar level of detail and information. Remember, the doctor is relying on us to provide the information about a situation so that he can figure out the best course of action. Even if there are further tests that can be run in the case of particular symptoms, a good account of your experiences may guide the decision about the best way to investigate further.

The Bottom Line

Since there are many complications either directly or indirectly linked to diabetes, this chapter is meant to serve as an overview of some of the most common ones. First and foremost, know that some of these complications can be detected early—before they become sympto-matic—with consistent monitoring and diligence. It is your job to make sure appointments are kept and tests are performed.

When you think you might be experiencing the symptoms of a new complication, check in with yourself and truly evaluate what is hap-pening physically, rather than allowing emotions of fear or denial to take over. Discuss your symptoms and concerns with your doctor in a thorough, thoughtful way and make sure that you are listened to. There are many, many ways to find relief from the discomfort caused by com-plications (as well as prevent them from getting worse) and your doc-tor should help you think outside the box, giving you tips to try at home and recommending (or at least answering your questions about) complementary and alternative therapies if there are some that might have a chance at helping you.

Be assertive. Get the help you need. Keep trying. Don't give up. Attain the highest quality of life that you can. Remember, complications aren't the end of the road—rather, think of them as new annoyances, hindrances or challenges to be dealt with . . . then deal with them.

4

Make Your Doctor Work for You

Over the course of 37 years with diabetes, I have had a number of doctors. Some good ones, a few great ones, and some downright miserable ones. It has taken me this long to put the right team together, but it is worth the effort that I put in. I am not sure where we got the idea that once we find a doctor willing to treat us that we should stick with him or her.

If your doctor doesn't stay on top of the changes in diabetes—you need to move on. If your doctor doesn't approach your care with the appreciation that *you* are really the one ultimately responsible for this disease and what it is doing to you, and that your health care providers are really there to assist and guide you to do the best you can—again, time to move on. (At this point, I imagine that some of you reading this think that I am nuts. I have heard so many people with type 2 diabetes tell me that their doctor will tell them when they need to change something in their treatment. Diabetes doesn't work that way—you can't pass the buck, as the buck stops with you. Always.)

When I was diagnosed in 1973, my care was transferred from my pediatrician to a cardiologist who treated adults. There were a couple of things wrong with this approach, the first being that I had diabetes, not heart problems, and the second being that I was 12 years old. Granted, there were no pediatric endocrinologists around, but this arrangement was setting me (and this doctor, for that matter) up to fail.

Somehow, my cardiologist guy and I mustered through several years together until I went to college. There it was determined by this guy that the main factor driving my out-of-control blood sugar levels was stress. After being yanked out of college for the first of several inpatient stays at a diabetes clinic, I followed the suggested "treatment strategy" and changed my major—not surprisingly, my blood glucose continued its wild swings, the implication being that it was my fault. Funny, while in the hospital, the doctors were not able to level out my blood sugar rollercoaster, despite their best efforts. However, as soon as I returned to the outside world, those same challenges went back to being my fault, according to them.

It should be noted that at this point in time, the only insulin in my treatment plan was NPH insulin, delivered in one whopping daily dose of 115 units. I would fill my syringe up to the 100 mark, then continue drawing the insulin in to "top it off," guessing at the last 15. This once a day "blast" of insulin was really the culprit in my inability to manage my blood sugar, but that was the approach to treating type 1 diabetes in those days. (Soon thereafter, the entry of other insulin onto the scene changed the picture of treatment for people with type 1 diabetes.)

I was anticipating great things when I located an endocrinologist associated with a hospital specializing in diabetes. At my first appointment, I launched into a fast-paced monologue chronicling the past few years—what I knew about my body, how it responded to treatment, all of the little tricks and work-arounds that I had developed to keep me functioning with diabetes on a daily basis. Without acknowledging anything, I had said in that half hour and with barely a glance, the doctor proceeded to pick up his calculator and use it to tell me what was wrong and what my correct dose should be—even facing the calculator toward me and pointing at the tiny display as "proof" that he was right.

Disappointed with this encounter but desperate, I followed the new treatment plan closely. Around this time, the A1c test came on the scene. My first results were impressive in that they were well into the double digits, providing concrete evidence that my blood glucose was wildly out of control and that no one was helping me—not my current doctor and certainly not his calculator.

Clearly, this was my disease and mine alone. I needed to choose the team of professionals that would help me—then I needed to lead that team. I would never again allow myself to be dictated to by a calculator that ignored the life lessons that I had accumulated.

Despite how much we may wish it was different, those of us with diabetes clearly require medical care. There are diagnostic tests to undergo, treatment options to pursue, complications and their symptoms to manage, and many other things that bring us into contact with doctors, nurses, and the medical system. Although a broken arm or strep throat can be adequately taken care of by someone you see once or twice and have no rapport with, diabetes is different. It is incurable. We will have diabetes for the rest of our lives, we therefore will need medical care for our diabetes for the rest of our lives. We will need different levels of support at different times.

The Real World

Diabetes is not curable. That means you'll be seeing some doctor for your diabetes for the rest of your life. Put in the time to make sure your doctors and other health care providers are the right ones for you.

It is crucial that we rise to the challenge of actively participating in our medical care. However, medical situations have an interesting effect on many of us. We might be powerhouses in the boardroom, people who do not hesitate to challenge our friends if we suspect an injustice, and/or parents who stop at nothing to ensure that we are getting the best for our children. However, when it comes to our own medical care, we tend to turn over more of ourselves to the doctor, participating less in medical decisions about our bodies than in discussions with waiters about how our meal is prepared.

To be involved in our medical care in a beneficial way, we need to get the following things in place: the right doctor for us, productive interactions with our doctors, the confidence and freedom to seek second opinions, and control over our medical information.

As a dear friend of mine who is a psychologist specializing in diabetes often reminds me, all aspects of health, including emotional health, are touched by this disease. It really takes a team to address them all adequately. However, even if you live in a place where there may only be one doctor with the expertise to treat diabetes, it is still possible to ensure that you are being heard and your questions are being answered.

Helping You Is Your Doctor's Job

I am not one of those angry patients who distrusts and reviles physician. I love the doctors that I have chosen to stay with as a patient, but it has been a process getting here. However, I can tell that many people have relationships with their doctors that are still a "work in progress," or that need to end altogether, indicated by the following remarks that I have heard:

> "I figure my doctor will tell me if I need to do something, so I don't pay attention to what my A1c result is."

> "When my doctor mentioned insulin for my type 2 diabetes, I decided to find another doctor who wouldn't insist on it."

> "I feel confused when I go to the doctor. I leave with half my questions unanswered and often don't even understand what he told me about my treatment plan."

We all have situations where we: nod our heads, even when we have no clue what is being said; accept something told to us, even if we know beyond a doubt that it is not true; and endure unfulfilling relationships. However, our interactions with our doctors should have *none* of those characteristics.

Take Charge

Your doctor works for *you*. Get your needs met and feel good about the relationship.

Find the Right Doctor for You

Take Charge

Evaluate your doctor situation: How did you end up with the doctor who is caring for your diabetes? Did you actively choose this doctor? Are you happy with him or her? What are the pros and cons of your current doctor?

Your experience with the doctor that diagnosed you was probably determined in part by the type of diabetes that you have and what your blood glucose levels were at that moment. Emotions, including sympathy, typically run high around a diagnosis of type 1 diabetes, especially in the very young. Pediatricians will usually quickly refer a child with extremely high blood glucose results first to the hospital and then to an endocrinologist or a colleague with more experience with pediatric diabetes.

On the other hand, the diagnosis of type 2 diabetes may be a longer, more drawn-out journey, beginning with the mention of "a little sugar" in the prediabetes stage and often including vague directives about diet and exercise. This may even culminate in threats about "the needle" if "bad habits" are not addressed. In other cases, it may be a symptom of a complication resulting from diabetes that has gone undiagnosed for years that brings you to a doctor in order to get the "double-whammy"—a diagnosis of a serious complication and the additional news that you also now have diabetes. This news is often accompanied by a bunch of "should haves" and "could haves."

Or, if you are fortunate, you may have experienced something different—a doctor who explains things clearly in a nonjudgmental manner, acknowledging your emotions and mapping out a logical, feasible treatment strategy. This wonderful doctor referred you to a certified diabetes educator to help you learn what you needed to know to stay healthy. This doctor has told you what you need to do in specific circumstances, like when you are sick or miss a dose of medication, as well as basic operating procedures of where to call after hours. You feel confident that you have a good partnership with this doctor—and that you can manage your diabetes for years to come with guidance from this particular person. Consider yourself lucky, as many, many people do not have this experience with the very people they are looking to for help and support to navigate their life with diabetes.

When a diagnosis of diabetes is made, people often feel very emotional and committed to the doctor that delivered the news, as well as overwhelmed and confused. The nature of many cases of diabetes is that they are unpredictable and act up sporadically, meaning that you may need to see the doctor very frequently for a while, then 6 months will go by where there is no need to see him. During these "quiet spells" it is easy to forget, or at least ignore, negative feelings about your doctor or the care that you are receiving (although, even if things seem "quiet," you need to keep up with your monitoring and treatment regimen, as well as see your doctors as scheduled).

Whether you just got diagnosed or you have been with one doctor for a long time, it is a good idea to take a long, hard look at your doctor. After all, you have not married this person or given birth to them (in most cases), so deciding that he or she is not the one for you is a relatively simple problem to fix.

Even if your current doctor is supposed to be the "diabetes king" in your area, it is no good if you feel worse than you did when you went in, because you were not listened to or taken seriously. I think most of us pretty much know how we feel about our current doctor on a gut level, but it wouldn't hurt to take a look at this list of questions and see how your doctor is doing:

- Does your doctor spend at least 15 minutes with you?

- When you ask about a new drug or possibly switching treatment, does your doctor listen, or does he dismiss the idea without giving a reason?

- Does your doctor spend time discussing your home glucose monitoring results or does he or she ignore them or talk about them in a vague, nonactionable way?

- Do you feel like your doctor adequately discusses the important things about new drugs (possible side effects, best results to expect, how long until the medication starts working) or symptoms that you might have (how bad it might get, different treatment options)?

- Are you treated with respect by the office staff, the nurses, and the doctor?

- When you tell your doctor about a new symptom, does he or she ever roll his or her eyes, tell you that what you are feeling is not possible or say anything else insensitive?

- Do you and your doctor actually discuss options for your treatment, or is it more a situation of being "told" by the doctor what the next steps are?

- How comfortable are you (or would you be) discussing a potentially embarrassing or confusing symptom with your doctor?

- Do you feel you can call your doctor to ask about side effects of drugs or new symptoms that you have without making an appointment?

- What does your "gut" say? Will this doctor be a good partner for you in the long-term?

- How accessible is your doctor by e-mail, text messaging, or telephone in case of an emergency? (This can be extremely important for a trip to the emergency room, as many of my friends with type 1 diabetes have told me horror stories of ER physicians "taking over" their diabetes care, over their protests, by removing CGMS and pump equipment or other dangerous things in the course of setting a broken bone or putting in stitches.)

The head of my medical team is probably the most incredible clinician I have ever met. He really understands diabetes. He is honest enough to tell me when there just isn't an answer—that sometimes it is just a diabetes thing that eludes explanation. He is always willing to listen and try different approaches. He is practical, acknowledging that his patients must be on board with his recommendations for there to be a chance of treatment working.

An example of my endocrinologist's understanding of how the whole person (in this case, me) has to be considered when treating this disease comes to mind. A few years ago, I experienced foot pain so severe that I was having trouble walking into town on Sunday mornings for breakfast, an activity I truly enjoy. I sought help in a local running store until I could get in to see my doctor. Upon examining my foot, my doctor explained why I was having the pain and we discussed a few options. When I asked him about trying a stabilizing running shoe instead of those "ugly diabetic shoes," he laughed and replied, "Why not try it? Even if it's not ideal, it will work better than if I convince you to get 'ugly shoes' that just sit in the back of your closet." Our compromise worked perfectly—I wear my running shoes every day for a couple of hours, allowing me to wear my favorite newest foot fashions the rest of the time.

The Real World

Remember, diabetes is more than daily challenges of managing blood glucose—which I must say, despite the number of years I have lived with diabetes, my levels still make sense only half of the time. There are many other things to monitor and manage. Can you talk about these symptoms with your doctor so that he or she understands what impact they really have on your life? Do you manage the treatment plan together to ensure the right tests and preventive steps are taken?

Know What You Want in a Doctor

Take Charge
You can't find the right doctor if you don't know what you want.

It is important that you know what you want in a doctor to help you manage your diabetes. Sure, a pretty waiting room with current issues of frivolous design and celebrity gossip magazines is always an asset. However, the relationship will go deeper than that, resulting in decisions that you have to adhere to and live with after you leave the office.

Take a couple of minutes and consider the following characteristics of what you might want in a doctor:

General practitioner or endocrinologist? Although most people with type 1 diabetes start seeing an endocrinologist soon after their diagnosis, the majority of people with type 2 diabetes remain under the care of a general practitioner/primary care physician. To evaluate if you should consider switching to an endocrinologist or adding one to your team, see the section "When is it time to move to an endocrinologist?" later in this chapter.

Does the doctor specialize in diabetes? Clearly, primary care physicians see everyone for everything, but even among endocrinologists, there are those that specialize only in the treatment of diabetes, while others treat many diseases of the endocrine system in addition to diabetes, such as hypothyroidism, adrenal disorders, and problems with sex hormones. The diabetes specialists have seen many more patients with diabetes and a much broader variety of complications, including rare ones. Although it is true that every case of diabetes is unique, doctors that see "all diabetes, all the time" are more likely to have seen situations very similar to yours. That will help them to predict what medication might be the most effective for you and what side effects you might experience.

Is the doctor affiliated with a diabetes clinic? If you are lucky enough to live within a reasonable distance to a diabetes clinic, you may want to give serious consideration to becoming a patient there. The benefits can be huge. The clinic may participate in a number of clinical trials and be aware of others that may be appropriate for you. Most likely, the diabetes center has strong relationships with the specialists and therapists that people with diabetes might need, even in obscure fields, such as: psychiatrists with experience with diabetes patients, retinologists, nephrologists, and others. In addition, the staff at diabetes clinics can often answer many of your questions over the phone. You can also be creative—if there is a diabetes clinic that is too far away to be your main source of medical care, you can try to find a local doctor that is willing to consult with the clinic, allowing you to go to the diabetes clinic once a year for a comprehensive evaluation.

What is the doctor's approach to managing diabetes and complications?

Some physicians like to leave big decisions, like which oral medications to try or if it might be time to start insulin therapy up to the patient. Others have very definite preferences for certain medications, to the point that they may be referred to as "the metformin guy" or "that Symlin doctor" and be very reluctant, or even unwilling, to prescribe anything else. Still others interview the patients at length about certain lifestyle factors, their expectations and fears, as well as their history. The doctor will then combine what the patient has told them with their experience with the various drugs in similar cases and make a recommendation based on all of these factors.

The Real World

Learn the "back story" to new treatments, especially before insisting that your doctor consider them in your case. The situation is usually more complex than you might think.

Also, some doctors will readily and happily send you to other professionals or therapists to solve a problem or manage a new issue. Others may wait until you ask to be referred. Some doctors take care of managing the integrated care, whereas others simply tell you what kind of specialist you need or give you a phone number and send you on your way. It pays to figure out what the ideal approach is for you— some of us would prefer to be told to go here at this time, whereas other people like to participate in researching other physicians and setting up their own appointments according to their schedules.

How aggressive do you want your doctor to be in your treatment? Decide if you are the type of person who wants to try the newest or the strongest approach to tightly controlling your blood glucose. Maybe you prefer a more conservative approach that reduces the risk of hypoglycemia. There isn't a universal correct answer here, but you should know which strategy you are the most comfortable with and make sure that your doctor is supportive of taking this route. (However, make sure that the decisions that you and your doctor make are based on results and not just convenience. There may be several different approaches to treatment that help you reach your target glucose goals—especially for people with type 2 diabetes—some easier to deal with than others. However, a doctor that does not use data to drive decisions or does not mention it when your glucose levels are far from your target because he or she is afraid of upsetting you or doesn't want to spend the time educating you is NOT acceptable.)

What are the doctor's research interests? Researchers are up-to-date on the latest treatments, at least the ones that they are looking at, but often have less time for patient interaction. However, if you have a specific complication or some aspect of diabetes that they are interested in, it might be a perfect fit.

Does board certification matter to you? You may wonder what the advantages to having a doctor who is board certified are. Here is the official answer from the Web site of the American Board of Medical Specialties (AMBS):

"If your doctor is certified by an ABMS Member Board, it means he or she is dedicated to providing exceptional patient care through a rigorous, voluntary commitment to lifelong learning through board certification and ABMS Maintenance of Certification (MOC). In addition to completing years of schooling, fulfilling residency requirements and passing the exams required to practice medicine in your state, your board certified specialist participates in an ongoing process of continuing education to keep current with the latest advances in medical science and technology in his or her specialty as well as best practices in patient safety, quality health care and creating a responsive patient-focused environment."

Personally, if I found a doctor I liked who wasn't board certified, I would not let that deter me from becoming her patient. However, I am happy with the knowledge that my endocrinologist is board certified. As people with diabetes, we are looking for doctors who are certified in endocrinology, diabetes, and metabolism by the American Board of Internal Medicine. If you are interested in checking out a specific neurologist, you can go to the Web site of ABMS (**www.abms.org**) and click on "Is Your Doctor Certified?" You will have to register, but the service is free of charge.

Does the doctor have Diabetes Registered Provider recognition? The American Diabetes Association has partnered with the National Committee for Quality Assurance to create a designation to recognize doctors who "use evidence-based measures and provide excellent care to their patients with diabetes." This program is called the Diabetes Recognition Program (DRP)—for doctors to get diabetes registered provider (DRP) recognition, they must complete a lengthy application, including submitting data from 25 patient charts for review. They must demonstrate that they have success in treating patients with diabetes, including meeting certain A1c targets, controlling blood pressure and LDL cholesterol, providing advice or treatment for smoking cessation and examining patients for diabetes complications involving kidneys, feet and eyes. You can find a physician with DRP recognition by going to recognition.ncqa.org and selecting "Diabetes Recognition Program" from the pull-down menu.

How open is the doctor (and how open are you) to complementary and alternative medicine? Studies show that many people with diabetes try some form of complementary and alternative medicine (CAM) to try to address blood glucose levels or discomfort from complications at some point after diagnosis. My guess is that most people don't tell their doctors some of the stuff they try, especially if it is really "out there." However, many doctors support the use of things like biofeedback, reiki, massage, and reflexology to alleviate symptoms or stress and most don't object to such noninvasive approaches (they may even be able to recommend practitioners who have experience with diabetes). However, if you are interested in some of the more potent herbal therapies (or, in my opinion, anything that you injest) or any of the more dramatic and potentially dangerous CAM modalities, you should make sure that you feel comfortable sharing these things with your doctor. There are many different ways that supplements or therapies can interact with what your doctor has prescribed for you and it is of utmost importance that he or she is aware of what is going on.

Make It Better

CAM treatments can be great for managing symptoms and just getting through the day. CAM, which includes things like yoga, acupuncture, vitamin supplements, and even prayer, can be just the thing to ease the discomfort of peripheral neuropathy or get a better night's sleep. You should be able to talk to your doctor about any CAM therapy you are considering or using.

Location and convenience are a consideration. Are you willing to drive a bit further to see a particular doctor? Does the doctor have appointments in the mornings or evenings? How long does it take to get an appointment? With what hospital is the doctor affiliated?

How to Find *Your* Doctor

Ask a person with diabetes. Ideally, you would know someone, or know someone who knows someone with diabetes (preferably the same type as you) who *loves* his or her doctor. If you are fresh out of personal contacts who also happen to have diabetes, support groups can be a great place for referrals. Once you know what you are looking for, you can talk to people at the support group and they will be happy to give you recommendations. This is an excellent place to get an honest appraisal of the doctors in your area.

Take Charge

Spend at least as much time checking out your doctor as you would a babysitter, your daughter's new boyfriend, a new employee, a lawyer, or an accountant.

Look for a Diabetes Registered Provider (DRP). As mentioned in the previous section, the American Diabetes Association and the National

Committee for Quality Assurance have a program to recognize doctors who demonstrate a commitment to providing excellent care for people with diabetes. These are doctors that have gone above and beyond sitting through the subject of diabetes in medical school—they have put real effort into getting the DRP designation. You can find a physician with DRP recognition by going to **recognition .ncqa.org** and selecting "Diabetes Recognition Program" from the pull-down menu.

Check out American Association for Clinical Endocrinologists. You can find an endocrinologist in your area who specializes in diabetes by going to **www.aace.com** and clicking on "Find an Endocrinologist" link under the "Resources" tab in the top menu.

Try putting a prospective doctor's name in PubMed. PubMed is the National Library of Medicine's database of medical research. Every article in almost every scientific medical journal is listed here. You can search a doctor's name by going to the site (**www.pubmed.gov**) and typing in the last name and the first initial (no commas) and the word *diabetes* into the search box. This will tell you about the diabetes-related research studies the doctor has been involved with.

Don't forget to call your insurance company. Once you have narrowed down the possibilities, you'll want to call your insurance company to make sure they will cover your office visits and treatments. Make sure that your provider is "in network" to save yourself money from extra charges.

Finally, interview a couple of doctors. Your first appointment with a new doctor is a time to interview and evaluate the doctor on the points that are important to you. Do not hesitate to ask as many questions as you want. Do not feel uncomfortable—after all, these are people who will eventually ask us about our sexual dysfunction, incontinence, and constipation—a couple of questions from us about appointment frequency and best ways to contact him in case of a weekend relapse should not rattle anyone too much. Make sure you get your questions answered: Is there a nurse on call? How often does he or she want to see you? Will he or she make a custom treatment plan for you? Can he or she help coordinate your treatment with other specialists? What does he or she think about alternative and complementary approaches?

Write your questions down before your appointment and assert yourself to make sure they all get answered. Ideally, you can take someone with you to take notes. If you can't, make sure to write down the answers to your questions, as we typically can only remember a small portion of what is said.

When Is It Time to Move to an Endocrinologist?

In contrast with the vast majority of people with type 1 diabetes, who have their diabetes treated by endocrinologists, most people who are diagnosed with type 2 diabetes are initially under the care of their general practitioner (GP) for some time. Although some GPs are extremely knowledgeable about diabetes and are really invested in their patients' treatment strategies, many do not have a great deal of enthusiasm for treating diabetes. There are several reasons for this, including: they lack the training needed to effectively create treatment plans, they are frequently disappointed with lack of patient adherence, they have neither the time nor resources needed to educate their patients and monitor their progress.

Patients often feel a loyalty to their GPs, but everyone needs to ask himself or herself if this doctor is the best he or she can do in terms of a partner to help him or her effectively manage his or her diabetes.

Here are some questions to ask yourself to decide if you should consider moving to an endocrinologist (or at least getting a second opinion):

- How comfortable is your doctor treating your diabetes? It is perfectly appropriate to ask your doctor this question, as well as follow-ups, such as: How many patients with diabetes are you currently treating? Are you usually pleased with their outcomes? Do you have relationships with appropriate specialists and other professionals that I will need to see (such as a retinologist and certified diabetes educator)? Do you have the time to teach me what I need to know and work with me to develop and monitor my treatment plan? Will you use my test results (A1c and blood glucose monitoring results) to make decisions, and will you push me when needed?

- Does your doctor spend time discussing your blood glucose monitoring results? Does he or she modify your treatment plan accordingly? Is he or she available for questions?

- Does your doctor do all of the things mentioned in the comprehensive diabetes evaluation on page 107?

- Are you having a hard time controlling your blood glucose as evidenced by your A1c and home monitoring results?

- Are you on a complicated treatment regimen of several different pills?

- Are you on insulin (or may be considering it)?

- Have you had a new complication while under the care of your current doctor? Is the doctor caring for this adequately or referring you to specialists for care?

- Have you been hospitalized for diabetic ketoacidosis (DKA) or hyperosmolar hyperglycemic noketotic syndrome (HHNS)?

- Have you been diagnosed with another health problem or have a situation that may make treating your diabetes more complicated (an autoimmune disease, pregnancy, cancer)?

- Is your current doctor resistant to your seeking second opinions? Does he or she try to handle everything himself or herself (as opposed to consulting endocrinologists or other specialists)?

If you answered "yes" to any of the questions previously, it may be time to see an endocrinologist. Depending on your situation, you may want to move all of your care to the endocrinologist. You could also see an endocrinologist for your diabetes care and have your current doctor continue to manage the rest of your care. Alternatively, you could see the endocrinologist for a consultation comprised of one or two visits, then return to your GP to implement the advice of the endocrinologist. Do not hesitate to ask for a referral to an endocrinologist if you think that would help you get the best care (for tips on how to ask for a second opinion, see page 117).

Certified Diabetes Educator: A Crucial Part of the Team

Even when you have found the *perfect* doctor, who knows *everything*, and whom you just *love*, your search is not over, because your team is not complete. As wonderful and fabulous and knowledgeable as your doctor may be, he or she will simply not have the time to help you learn everything that you need to master to manage your diabetes. Managing diabetes really, really requires our participation to have the best possible outcomes. However, not only is there an enormous amount of information that one has to absorb, a person with diabetes quickly has to learn how to operationalize that information and use it in real life, tweaking and strategizing along the way.

This is where the certified diabetes educator (CDE) comes in. A CDE is someone who has met certain requirements and has at least 1000 hours of direct experience educating people with diabetes. They can be any of several different professions, including: nurses, doctors, psychologists, dietitians, pharmacists, and others. According to the American Association of Diabetes Educators, CDEs focus on helping people with the following self-care behaviors: "healthy eating, being active, monitoring blood glucose, taking medication, problem solving, healthy coping and reducing risks."[1]

CDEs work in various settings. It is possible that your clinic has a CDE on staff, if it is a specialized facility treating diabetes. They also work from hospitals, other clinics, or other settings. It is ideal if your doctor has a CDE (or several) that he works with and trusts that he can refer you to. Otherwise, you can find a CDE in your area by going to the Web site of the American Association of Diabetes Educators at **diabeteseducator.org**, and clicking on the "Find a Diabetes Educator" link under the "About Diabetes Education" header.

How often you see a CDE depends on many things. Surely, most people newly diagnosed with diabetes will want to go to a CDE. After that, some people go quarterly or to as many sessions as their insurance will pay for, until they feel like they have enough information. Others go when they make a big change, like adding insulin into their treatment plan or seriously considering pregnancy, while still other people visit their CDE to help them figure out a longer-term strategy for starting and maintaining an exercise program.

Many people visit a CDE immediately following their diagnosis with diabetes, then never go again. This is not such a great strategy. CDEs can help you troubleshoot and assimilate all the information into your real-life situation. Also, there are so many things happening in diabetes—new technologies, improved meds, better ways to address some of the discomforts that we encounter—many of which doctors

don't know about. CDEs can help us stay up-to-date with current inno-
vations to help us manage diabetes.

Components of the Comprehensive Diabetes Evaluation

As we know, diabetes is a complicated disease that requires thorough
monitoring by doctors—this goes far beyond a semiannual or quarterly
A1c and the occasional prescription. In terms of controlling blood glucose and assessing complications, your doctor needs to know where you
are at the moment he or she is seeing you, evaluate how you have been
doing since he or she last saw you, and determine how to proceed to try
to reduce the risk of complications and manage the ones that come
along. To do this effectively, he or she needs to gather lots of information—going far beyond asking "how's it been going?" You may be seeing
different kinds of doctors—if you have type 1 diabetes, you are likely
under the care of an endocrinologist, and if you have type 2 diabetes,
your primary care physician may be treating your diabetes. Regardless of
your doctor's specialty, he or she should be aware of specific things about
your health (or at least make sure that another doctor is monitoring that
aspect of your diabetes). Here is a list of the "Components of the comprehensive diabetes evaluation" adapted from the American Diabetes Association's *2010 Standards of Medical Care in Diabetes*:

Medical History

The first time you give your medical history to a new doctor may take
some time, as your doctor will want to know all about your diabetes
diagnosis, including how old you were at the time and what circumstances led to your diagnosis (DKA, routine blood work turning up a
high blood glucose level, etc.). Of course, he will also want to know
your full medical history, including everything about your health that is
related, directly or indirectly, to diabetes, such as history of complications and other health problems that you may have. You will also be
asked questions about the following:

- Eating patterns and nutritional status
- Weight history
- Current and past physical activity levels
- Any diabetes education have you received in the past

- Children and adolescents (or their parents) will be asked about growth and development history
- All previous treatment regimens and how you responded to them, including A1c records from this time

Current Treatment of Diabetes

Your doctor will want to go over your current treatment plan and how you are responding to it, including:

- Medications that you are currently taking
- Any food plans that you are following
- Physical activity patterns (kind of exercise, frequency, intensity)
- Results of home glucose monitoring and how you are using the data (the doctor should review blood glucose results from your monitor or log book, rather than just asking, "How has your blood glucose been?")

Acute Problems and Long-term Complications

The doctor will be very interested in any diabetes-related problems you are having around controlling your blood glucose or possible or confirmed complications. Make sure that you include everything that has happened since you last saw the doctor—don't forget emergency room visits or information from appointments with other doctors, including:

- Hypoglycemic episodes (how severe they were, how frequent have they been, what caused them or circumstances surrounding the episodes, and what symptoms you experienced)
- DKA (frequency, severity, and cause or circumstances)
- Any complications that you have experienced since you last saw the doctor and status of existing complications, including: diabetic retinopathy, kidney problems, foot injuries, peripheral neuropathy, gastroparesis, sexual dysfunction, heart problems, peripheral artery disease
- Any psychosocial challenges that you are experiencing

- Any overall changes that you are experiencing in things like sleep patterns, appetite, energy levels, and so forth
- Any dental disease or problems

Physical Examination

The doctor will conduct a physical exam (although the nurse might collect some of the data), including:

- Weight and BMI (body mass index)
- Blood pressure measurement, maybe taking measurements when you are laying down then change positions to sitting or standing
- Examining the eyes with an ophthalmoscope, which is a hand-held instrument with a light (Note: this is not a substitute for an exam by an opthalmologist or retinologist)
- Thyroid palpation
- Thorough skin examination, looking for acanthosis nigricans (a skin disorder characterized by dark, thick, velvety skin in body folds and creases) and taking a look at insulin injection sites
- Comprehensive foot examination, including: thorough inspection of the skin on the foot, including between the toes; palpating the foot for pulses that can be felt in your feet (to see how well your circulation is working in your lower extremities); testing reflexes in the feet; testing sensation in the feet using a tuning fork, sharp/dull instruments and a monofilament

Laboratory Evaluation

The following lab tests will be run annually (except A1c, which will be more frequent):

- A1c (every 3–6 months, depending on type of diabetes and other factors)
- Fasting lipid panel, including total cholesterol, LDL and HDL, and triglycerides

- Liver function tests
- Test for urine albumin excretion with spot urine albumin/ creatinine ratio
- Serum creatinine and calculated GFR
- Thyroid levels in type 1 diabetes, dyslipidemia, or women older than 50 years of age

Referrals

The doctor will also ask you about the following exams or visits, providing referrals to specialists where necessary:

- Annual dilated eye exam
- Family planning and gynecological exam for women
- Registered dietitian for medical nutritional therapy (food and meal planning)
- Diabetes self-management education through classes or individual visits with a certified diabetes educator (CDE)
- Dental exam
- Appointment with a mental health professional, if needed

Your doctor should be aware of how you are doing in each of the previously mentioned areas. Of course, your exams will be individualized to fit your situation—an exam of a person who has been living with type 1 diabetes since childhood (who is already under the care of a retinologist, gastroenterologist and a cardiologist for monitoring and to manage any potential complications) will be much different than the exam for a person newly diagnosed with type 2 diabetes who has not yet started treatment or been thoroughly evaluated for complications. Regardless of your health and diabetes status, it is important to be aware of all of the things that go into monitoring the health of a person with diabetes—if your doctor does not do a certain test or seem interested in what you have to say, speak up.

Have a Productive Conversation With Your Doctor

Doctors have a way of unsettling people. Lawyers, CEOs, and senators lose their bravado and self-confidence when it comes to talking with doctors. Psychologically, we are vulnerable when we are discussing our own health. Intellectually, we don't have the same mastery of the terminology that the doctor has. Physically, we may be sitting in a paper robe with (or without) ties in the back. All of these factors can result in us feeling flustered and nervous during conversations with our doctors—times when we really need to be communicating well and remembering details.

Many people with diabetes, especially those with type 2 diabetes who were diagnosed later in life and have not had to grapple with a chronic illness before, take a more passive role in their care, waiting for the doctor to tell them what the plan is, when it is time to make a change. These people may rely on the doctor to tell them how they are doing and even how they are feeling, instead of really thinking through how everything fits together and what is not working for them.

Take Charge

Prepare for your doctor's visit as if it were a job interview or a major presentation. Think about it ahead of time, visualize the visit, and set goals.

By preparing for your doctors' visits and making a few shifts in your attitude about all things medical, you'll get a lot more out of your medical care. You won't leave confused or with unanswered questions, and you will establish a true partnership with your doctor. Good communication and rapport with your doctor is a key component in your medical care. Having a good relationship with the right doctor can speed diagnosis and treatment as well as reduce a tremendous amount of the stress that surrounds diabetes.

Be an active patient. Studies have shown that "active patients"—patients that ask questions—like their doctors better. The studies also show that doctors like these patients better. At first you might think that the doctors would find these patients to be annoying. Think about it a little more. Imagine you are a doctor, facing exam room after exam room of patients every day. Each room contains a passive patient who just answers your questions and is intimated by you. Now, put a patient in one room who is determined to feel better, who asks intelligent questions, and with whom you can share some of your knowledge. That visit is much more exciting and rewarding. You can be that exceptional patient by being curious about your health and diabetes. Remember, doctors became doctors because they find health (and maybe diabetes) fascinating. Share that fascination, ask some questions, and be an "active patient."

Recently I was reviewing some research that showed that during the typical doctor visit, the doctor did most of the talking. It seems like an active patient will talk at least as much as the doctor, in a give-and-take exchange.

Tell your doctor what kind of patient you are. Everyone with diabetes is different. Some of us want to "grab the bull by the horns" and do everything we can all at once to manage this disease, regardless of cost or discomfort. Other people are overwhelmed at the beginning and want to try less drastic measures while they learn about their new diagnosis. It is important to convey to the doctor where you fall on the spectrum of aggressive versus conservative approaches.

The Real World

You have only one primary diabetes doctor, but that doctor has hundreds of patients. Be unique, be memorable. Be that patient that your doctor thinks about after you leave and does a little bit of "extra research" to help.

Doctors usually treat people based on their experience with other patients. Every doctor has hundreds of patients he or she sees, and unless you tell the doctor otherwise, he or she will assume that you are more or less like his or her other patients. This is normal—doctors don't automatically know your dreams, plans, tolerance level for pain and inconvenience, willingness to experiment with different approaches. It helps if you condense your feelings about some of these things into a paragraph and tell your doctor exactly what kind of patient you are.

Prepare for your appointment. We've talked about your attitude toward your doctor, now it is time to focus on action. Treat your doctor's appointments like important business meetings—prepare for them. You probably would have a list of questions ready before going to see any other professionals (an accountant, a lawyer, a realtor), and it just makes sense to get your thoughts and questions organized before seeing your doctor.

Don't think that you are overstepping your boundaries—it is respectful to come prepared to an appointment. Make a pledge to yourself to do this before every doctor's appointment. Here are some suggestions for getting prepared:

Step 1: Update your doctor. Write out a few bullet points that summarize how you feel and what is happening. Refer to "How to talk to your doctor about your symptoms" from Chapter 3 to make sure that you include relevant information about how your symptoms are affecting you. Be short and to the point, but don't leave out anything that might be important. Be sure to include any lifestyle adjustments you are making, including changes in diet, exercise, and supplements. Also, let your doctor know about any alternative providers you are seeing, such as acupuncturists, chiropractors, and massage therapists.

Step 2: Decide what you want to improve. Make a list of anything about your health that you want to improve. You may be surprised what can happen if you just ask. For example, if you have headaches when you wake up or symptoms of hypoglycemia several hours after you finish exercising, your doctor will be able to suggest changes to your medication dosages, timing, or suggest how to add in snacks—all of which can make a big difference. Mention what you would like to improve and see if your doctor can help.

Step 3: List any additional questions. You may have heard the adage that "there is no such thing as a stupid question." While I don't believe that is true in every situation, I believe that there is no question about your health that you should be afraid to ask your doctor. They can range from the insignificant-to-most-people-but-a-big-deal-to-you (ie, Will Glucophage help my acne?) to the improbable, but still of concern (ie, Can the artificial sweeteners in diet soda cause cancer?). List them all. Then, most importantly, *ask* them all.

Understand your doctor's role. Make sure that you are satisfied in terms of quality of medical care—however, don't expect too much or the wrong things from your doctor. His or her role in your medical care is just that—the medical side of things. Usually, your doctor is not trained in behavior change, stress reduction, or counseling. Your doctor may or may not know details about alternative therapies. Expect your doctor to know everything about interpreting the results diagnostic tests, the medical aspects of your diabetes, and your treatment. You can ask about the other things, but your doctor may or may not have the answers for you. You may need to find a few other professionals to help you with the in-depth information that you want.

The Real World

Be fair with your doctor. The best doctor is the one who says, "I don't know," and refers you to someone else for a particular complication when he or she can't manage it himself or herself. You wouldn't go to a divorce lawyer for your corporate merger and you shouldn't expect your diabetes doctor to be able to handle everything.

Take notes. Don't trust yourself to remember everything the doctor says. Jot down key terms and ask the doctor to spell them if you need to.

Don't forget nurses. You may spend more time with the nurses than with the doctor. You can ask a lot of questions while he or she is taking your vital signs. Nurses often have a little bit more time than the doctor and may go into greater detail with you. This is especially true around "self-care" or personal maintenance tips, like instructions for giving yourself an injection or how to stay adherent to your medications.

Bring someone with you. That other person can be your notetaker and can remind you of questions that you have. Most importantly, the other person can help you to understand better and recall more accurately what the doctor has said. Also, having someone else along may help you find the resolve to stick to your list and ask all of your questions.

If you think of something you forgot to ask the doctor during your appointment, call the office and ask to talk to a nurse. The nurse can usually answer your question or find out the answer for you and call you back. Don't think that you are bothering the staff—they are there to help you, but it is your job to be precise and concise to make the phone calls efficient for them.

Get Some Plans in Place With Your Doctor

Many of us are reluctant to call our doctor's office with questions and concerns. We try to manage seemingly "little things" ourselves, only to find that the little things become bigger things and we end up in the doctor's office anyway with a more urgent situation. It is best to plan ahead and have a strategy on how different situations will be dealt with, rather than "reinventing the wheel" every time something happens. Never, I repeat, NEVER, worry that you are calling your doctor's office too much or that your questions are too trivial. This is your health, and your doctor should appreciate the active role that you are taking if you call for direction, rather than ignoring the problem or trying to figure things out yourself because you don't want to annoy anyone.

Planning Ahead

Doctors differ in their approach to patient care, often depending on the individual and their specific situation. Make sure you ask the doctor the following questions, as well as any others you can think of:

- What numbers on my glucose monitor should trigger a call to you (and what number should I call)—what is too high? Too low?

- How often do you recommend that I check my blood glucose and at what times of day? How would you prefer to review my results—directly from my monitor or from a log book?

- Should I call every time I am hypoglycemic or just when I have certain symptoms or frequency?

- When should I check for ketones? What should I do if they are positive (or at what levels should I take action)?

- What should I do if I can't reach you for diabetes-related problems?

- Which hospital should I go to for emergency care?

When to Call

There are some times when your doctor will definitely want to hear from you. These may include the following situations, but you will want to clarify these with your doctor to know his or her specific approach:

- When you are running a fever for more than 8 hours
- You are unable to eat for more than 6 hours
- You are vomiting and cannot hold down food for more than 6 hours
- You have had diarrhea for more than 6 hours
- You have run out of medication
- Your blood glucose will not go below 240 mg/dL for 24 hours or you have two readings of 300 mg/dL in a row (especially if you have type 2 diabetes)
- You think you have symptoms of DKA or HHNS (see Chapter 3)
- Your ketone levels are moderate or severe
- You have forgotten to take medication and you don't know what to do

Sick Day Plan

Everyone gets sick—colds, flu, stomach bugs. For people with diabetes, these routine illnesses can make things more challenging in terms of controlling blood glucose. Fever and infections can cause blood sugar to spike. Vomiting and diarrhea can upset the delicate balance among your medications, your food intake and your blood glucose levels, as well as cause dehydration, which is potentially very dangerous to people with diabetes. It is important to work with your doctor or CDE to know how to deal with each situation. Most likely, your sick day plan will include instructions like the following:

- Increase fluid intake (find out how much fluid per hour)
- Monitor blood glucose more frequently (find out how often)
- Specific blood glucose numbers that will prompt action
- How to adjust medication dosages, depending on the situation (get specific instructions)

- Which foods to eat in different situations
- Which over-the-counter medications are safe to take
- Begin monitoring ketones (certain people)
- When to call the doctor

Make sure your sick day plan has the phone numbers that you will need, including your doctor and where to call off-hours, as well as specific friends or family members that you could call if you have an emergency or just need help getting to the doctor or pharmacy.

Don't Be Afraid to Get a Second Opinion

The Real World

Doctors are people, people who can make honest mistakes. For big decisions, it just makes sense to get a second opinion if things are not 100% clear. Don't let feelings of loyalty or worries about offending a doctor get in the way of confirming a decision.

Why People Get Second Opinions

There are many reasons that you might want to get a second opinion on a specific complication or in the overall management of your diabetes. You may have started thinking about a second opinion after having thoughts similar to some of these:

"There must be better options for treating this." You tried, you really tried to make a go of it with the oral medication that your doctor prescribed. However, the side effects were terrible and you want to try something else. Your doctor says this is the best he or she can do for you. Maybe someone else has other ideas.

Take Charge

Your health is *yours*. Make your medical care *yours*, too.

"I would like to get the opinion of someone with more experience with my situation." Maybe, in addition to diabetes, you have another condition that requires you to take medications (such as corticosteroids) that send your blood glucose levels out of control. Maybe you are a woman with type 1 diabetes who wants to try to get pregnant using in-vitro fertilization, but your doctor is unsure how the hormone treatments will affect blood glucose levels. In either case, you would like to be seen by someone who has handled similar cases—or at least get their opinion. If you like this new doctor, it is possible that the "second opinion" will turn into a "referral," meaning that the new doctor will take over this part of your care.

Feel Confident in Your Decision to Seek a Second Opinion

There are many people out there who feel like they are cheating on their doctor when they seek a second opinion. I know it can be an awkward situation, unless your doctor brings it up himself or herself. However, most doctors will be happy for you to seek a second opinion, as it will probably make you more comfortable with your final decision and even more adherent to the treatment prescribed.

I am not promising that your doctor will have a positive reaction. Occasionally, doctors get angry, feeling like the patient doesn't trust their judgment or is searching for something specific that the current doctor doesn't agree with.

Script for Asking Your Doctor About a Second Opinion

Okay, it is one thing to keep telling you that it is your right to get a second opinion and that you have nothing to be nervous about. Clearly, however, you are the one who has to discuss it with your doctor and there may not be someone there with you in the situation, giving you a "thumbs-up" sign and whispering, "You go, girl (or boy)." So, here's a little script to adapt and practice before you go.

Try something like this:

> "This is a big deal to me and having another person weigh in would really increase my comfort level with any decisions. [Optional: Is there anyone you would recommend to help us with this specific problem?]"

Going in prepared with something like this may prevent you from blurting out something unfortunate in an emotional moment. Even if you are pretty sure that you are done with your doctor or that his or her decisions are not the right ones for you, getting upset or making accusations is just not productive.

Ways to Optimize Your Second Opinion

Gather all of your own medical records and get them to the other doctor in advance. This includes doctor's notes and any test results.

Make sure you get a report on the second doctor's findings. The new doctor might not communicate with your primary doctor (although they are supposed to). In addition, you will want this report for your records as well to use to conduct any of your own research on the topic.

Make sure the second doctor is board certified in the appropriate specialization. If you are going to go to the trouble of getting a second opinion, it is wise to go to someone who is up on the "latest and greatest" in their field. If you are seeking advice on an diabetes-specific problem, find someone board certified in endocrinology. If, however, you are looking for answers to problems around certain symptoms, find someone certified in that field. For instance, for help with heart issues, you would seek a doctor with certification in cardiology.

Make sure your insurance will pay. In some cases, especially when surgery or less common treatments are going to be tried, insurance companies will require a second opinion to verify the benefit to the patient and that it is indicated for the condition before they will agree to pay for the treatment or procedure. In other cases, insurance will not pay for a second opinion. Give your insurance company a call to find out.

What If Doctors Disagree?

There will be times when your doctors have different opinions. Make sure that you ask specific questions about why they came to the conclusions they did. What evidence did they have? Why does one think a certain medication is better than another for you? It may be that one doctor is relying solely on studies published in medical journals or how they "always" do things, while another doctor is basing his recommendations on what you have told him or her about yourself and how you have responded to treatments in the past. It is never a bad idea to do a

little of your own research on your condition, including even seeking a
third opinion, before making a decision. In the end, however, you may
have to "go with your gut" when choosing among treatment options or
which diagnosis to believe.

Take Charge

Ultimately, *you* will make the decisions about your health care.
Be prepared and know what you are doing.

Tame Your Medical Information

Take Charge

Don't expect your doctors to read your full medical chart at every
visit or to remember what happened to you a year ago. It is your
job to keep track of everything and remind your doctor of the
specifics of your situation.

An important part of actively participating in your medical care is having control over the huge amount of information about your situation.
Clearly, medical information can get out of control pretty quickly, especially with a chronic and complicated condition like diabetes. There is
information about doctors, procedures, tests, medications, billing, and
insurance. By having a system to collect and organize all of your health-
related information, you will be able to find what you need, when you
need it. Having all this information in one place will really help. When
you have an acute problem, are feeling sick, or are panicking about a
sudden new symptom, you are very likely to forget some important
details. These details could prevent potentially harmful drug interactions or may be used to speed diagnosis. Taking the time to gather your
information now will make you feel more in control of your diabetes
and more ready to deal with any health-related situation that may occur.

When I was preparing to see yet another endocrinologist in my
quest for quality care (who actually ended up being the one that I stuck
with for my care), I decided to write down a "history" of my diabetes to
give the new doctor as many pieces of the puzzle as I could. What
seemed like a straightforward task at the beginning proved to be

extremely challenging. To get even close to a complete account took not only hours of me searching my memory, but required the input of many other friends and family members—my brother, my partner, my closest friend and others. Each of these people was present and involved in my life during different phases of my diabetes and different struggles with complications. My psychologist friend reminded me that my "journey" with diabetes was not only about medical symptoms and treatments, and suggested I add in some emotional aspects and behavior into the story. My diabetes timeline took a great deal of effort, but paid off greatly in establishing a relationship with the wonderful doctor who is my current endocrinologist.

It's not really that fun to do this, but you will feel proud when you get this together. I recommend really trying to keep this current by making entries after each doctor appointment or major life event—at least update it annually. My diabetes history turned out to be such a huge volume of work that I was tempted to give it a snappy title, such as *Lost in the Islets of Langerhans: Lynn's Adventures with Diabetes.*

Step 1: ***Create a medical information binder.*** Get a binder to store your medical information in. Make sure it is one that will be comfortable (and fashionable) enough to carry to appointments.

Step 2: ***Decide on your emergency contact people.*** Label your first page "Emergency Contacts." Choose three people as your emergency contact people. They should be local and able to get to a hospital and help you if you need it. Be sure to tell each person that you are listing him or her as an emergency contact. Double-check phone numbers and other information. This is important; you will need this information handy when you go to see new doctors or if you are admitted to the hospital, in many cases. While you are at it, enter their phone numbers in your cell phone using the names "ICE1," "ICE2" and "ICE3" ("in case of emergency"), as police and paramedics often look for this.

Step 3: ***Write down your current doctors.*** Label the next page "My Doctors." Make a list of all your current doctors and medical providers, along with their telephone numbers and addresses. Be sure to list your doctors, including: your endocrinologist, primary care physician, gynecologist, cardiologist, podiatrist, dentist, eye doctor and any other service providers like physical therapists. This is also a good place to list the numbers of your pharmacies, including the mail-order one that provides your insulin or specialty drugs.

Step 4: ***Write down your current diagnoses.*** Title the next page "Diagnoses/Conditions/Complications." In addition to your diabetes, list any medical conditions that you have been diagnosed with. Include things like high blood pressure and high cholesterol, as well as any allergies or illnesses. Try to recall the date of diagnosis. You can estimate if you have to. Give some indication of your status by using words like "mild," "under control" or "severe."

Step 5: ***Write down your current medications.*** This one is very important. Label the page "Current Medications" and list all the medications you are currently taking and what they are for. List both the commercial and drug names of the medication. Be sure to include the dosage and the number of times a day you take it. Estimate when you first started taking each drug and if (and when) the dosage was changed.

Step 6: ***Write down anything else you are taking.*** Label this page "Non-Prescription Items." If you are taking any vitamins or other supplements, include the name, dosage, and frequency just like you did with your medications. You may also describe what the supplement is for and/or what the main ingredients are. Also include nonprescription drugs, such as cold remedies, pain relievers, laxatives, or stool softeners—anything that you take without a prescription. If you are trying any complementary and alternative medicine approaches, make a note of these, especially things like chelation, bee venom therapy, homeopathic remedies, or anything else that enters your body.

Take Charge

You think more about your health than your doctor does. Keep track of your thoughts, health events, and other medical details.

Step 7: ***Record your medical events.*** Make a separate page for each time you had a serious medical event, such as a surgery, a hospitalization, a prolonged course of treatment, labeled with a reference to that event (for example, "2004 Treatment for Retinopathy" or "2006 Hospitalization for Ketoacidosis"). On these pages, write down any information related to the event: symptoms, diagnosis, date, treating physician, treatment, outcome, medications, dosage, side effects, tests run, results. Record as many of the details as you can. Be sure to include any related test results on your form and include a copy of them in your binder if you have them.

Step 8: ***Record your past stressors.*** Only after I did this myself, upon the recommendation of my psychologist friend, did I see why this was a useful component of my medical history and information. Many major life events are caused by or impact your diabetes—maybe you quit your job because it was too stressful at a time when you were experiencing a complication, maybe the death of a family member corresponds with some high A1c results, maybe you gained better control over (or lost control of) your blood glucose after you got married. Label this sheet "Life Events" and list as many of these moments as you can, with approximate dates.

Step 9: ***Get a box and label it "Medical Information."*** Whenever you receive a benefits statement in the mail, billing information, or any other piece of paper about your medical management and care, put it in the box. That way you know where everything is. If you need something, you can sort through the box until you find it. It is not an elegant solution, but it will work because it is convenient to do. This is for information that you should save but probably won't need access to. Be sure that test results are placed in your binder immediately—don't put them into your box.

Step 10: Keep your binder current. Don't forget to update your information whenever anything changes. Keep your emergency contacts, test results, current medications, information about your doctors, as well as any other relevant information up-to-date.

Tips for Making Your Medical Information Binder Complete and Useful

Go electronic. You could also do all of this electronically, if that is more your style. Some people find it much easier to keep their medical information current if they can enter it into a computer. Most labs and clinics will scan and e-mail test results and other reports if you request this.

Don't rely only on your memory. Ask friends and family to help you recall dates, medications and procedure names. You may need to talk with your doctor or a nurse to complete the task. Just call the office and ask when a good time would be to call back and get some information from your chart. You can also ask for a copy of your medical records, though a nurse may be able to find the information faster than you— she may also be able to read your doctor's handwriting.

The Bottom Line

Your medical care can only be as good as your relationship with your doctor. A good patient-doctor partnership can open up new possibilities for really honing in on the main health concerns that you have and collaborating with your doctor to tackle them strategically, tweaking things as you go along, until the best solution is discovered. However, a bad relationship (or even a neutral one) may lead to important things being overlooked, misdiagnosed, untreated or not taken seriously. This results in frustration and, ultimately, unnecessary suffering on your part.

In his book, *How Doctors Think*, Jerome Groopman reveals some astounding things about the thought processes of physicians. The most interesting from the viewpoint of the patient is that doctors' thinking is not simply a computer-like process of taking in data and spitting out diagnoses and treatment plans. Nope, as it turns out, doctors are people. And just like other people, doctors are influenced by their emotions, including their feelings about their patients and their interactions with them. This is where we come in. Let's face it, doctors cannot be expected to care more about our health and our symptoms than we do.

To that end, we have to step up and show that we are ready to do the work to hold up our end of the partnership. We have to be interested enough in our care to come prepared to appointments with questions, observations, and goals. We have to be thoughtful enough about our symptoms to put the effort in to really think about them in specific terms and be able to give this information to the doctor. To get the best care possible, the care that we deserve, we need to be active, interested patients—the very kind of patients that got many doctors excited about going into medicine to help people.

5

Help Treatment Help You

Let me start by saying that I am grateful that I am writing this chapter now, and not 37 years ago when I was first diagnosed with type 1 diabetes and the best treatment available to me was what would now be considered a barbaric once-a-day dose of neutral protamine Hagedorn (NPH) insulin. Treatment and other tools to manage your diabetes have come so far since that time. People diagnosed with type 1 and type 2 diabetes now have a realistic shot at achieving pretty stable blood glucose control, as opposed to the wild swings that I endured and the barbaric practice of doctors using hypoglycemic insulin reactions to indicate if your dosage was correct—if you didn't have enough "hypos," you were considered not to be getting enough insulin and the dose was increased.

However, I am also not going to tell you that everything is rosy and life with diabetes is now carefree, thanks to all of the wonderful progress that has been made. That is not the case, not by a long shot. Arriving at just the right dosages of just the right medications is often a matter of trial and error. Then it seems that not long after this perfect algorithm is discovered, something in your body changes (hormones change, natural insulin production decreases, you lose weight, you gain weight) and you and your doctor have to start tinkering again with your meds. On top of everything often comes the implication that the medications would work better if you were doing better at dealing with your diabetes. Put this all together, and treatment for diabetes is a big, confusing, constantly shifting challenge that some people find overwhelming or not worth the effort. They may be lax about sticking to their treatment regimen or give up altogether.

Regardless of your situation, there is no doubt that decisions around treatment, both drugs to control glucose and medications and procedures to treat or manage complications, can be emotionally charged and filled with questions and uncertainties. By learning to take charge of your treatment decisions, you will find the solution that is right for you, resulting in better adherence and confidence in your chosen plan of attack.

Consider All Aspects of Treatment

Although it would be great if one of the treatments for diabetes had a huge margin of advantages over the other drugs in all aspects, this is often not the case for every patient. Like everyone else with diabetes seems to be, your decision around treatment should take into account a bunch of complicated factors and may require a little research on your part.

Make It Better

Don't neglect your emotions and financial situation when choosing a therapy. Your treatment choice needs to be the best fit for you and your lifestyle, not just what might look like a better option according to a research study. However, don't let finances be an excuse to getting adequate treatment—there are usually ways to afford the best treatment for you. Put some time into investigating these options before writing something off as "too expensive."

Treatment Overview*

The goal of this section is not to offer a comprehensive guide to diabetes medications. Rather, it is to provide a glimpse of what kinds of drugs are out there and what the mechanisms of action are for these drugs, so that you can use this as a starting place to begin your own research or understand a little more about your doctor's treatment strategy.

---

* Disclaimer: As Lynn works in the pharmaceutical industry, all descriptions of specific medication were written entirely by Dr. Stachowiak to avoid any potential conflict of interest.

In general, there are fundamental differences in treating people with type 1 diabetes and type 2 diabetes, as many people with type 2 diabetes are still making some insulin, whereas people with type 1 diabetes cease making insulin within a couple of years after diagnosis. Therefore, especially in the early stages, many people with type 2 diabetes are treated with medications to work with the insulin that their bodies are producing, whereas people with type 1 diabetes get all of their insulin from the outside. However, some people with type 2 diabetes eventually need insulin and their treatment regimens may closely resemble those prescribed for type 1 individuals.

Insulin

There are many types of insulin, which are designed to take effect at different rates and last for different durations. There are short- and rapid-acting versions, insulin designed to last overnight, 24-hour insulin, and intermediate options. It is likely that your doctor will prescribe a combination of these different types to suit your lifestyle and provide the best possible glucose control. (Note: If you have type 1 diabetes and your doctor only prescribes a long-acting insulin, it might be time to seek a second opinion, unless you are in the short-lived "honeymoon" period that some people experience immediately after diagnosis. Although people with type 2 diabetes often start their insulin therapy with just a basal, or long-acting, insulin, this is not the standard of care for people with type 1 diabetes. The only people with type 1 diabetes who are using just one type of insulin are on insulin pumps.)

Rapid-acting insulin, such as Humalog (lispro), Novolog (aspart), and Apidra (glulisine), start working within 5 to 15 minutes. They reach their peak action from 30 minutes to 3 hours and last for 3 to 5 hours. Short-acting insulin (humulin or novolin), which is known as "regular" insulin, starts acting within an hour. It peaks within 2 to 4 hours and lasts for 6 to 8 hours. Intermediate insulin, NPH, starts working within 2 hours, peaks between 6 to 10 hours and lasts for up to 16 hours. The long-acting insulin, such as Lantus (glargine) and Levemir (detemir), start working within 1 to 2 hours and last for approximately 24 hours with no peak action. The idea behind all of these different types of insulin is to simulate how your pancreas works—there is always a little insulin circulating in the bloodstream, with the pancreas releasing large "boluses" in response to ingested food.

All of the insulin varieties that are currently available must be injected or delivered through an insulin pump. The injections are given with a syringe or an insulin pen, which is basically a prefilled syringe that can be dialed to the correct dosage. Many people want to know why insulin cannot be taken as a pill or liquid. Insulin is a protein and, at least in current formulations, is digested by stomach acid and rendered ineffective. However, at the time of this writing, there are currently a couple of companies with oral insulin (spray or capsules) in clinical trials, as well as an inhaled version coming to market.

Many people with type 1 diabetes swear by (and sometimes at) their insulin pumps. These are devices that deliver appropriate amounts of rapid-acting insulin around the clock—tiny and frequent amounts to maintain your basal rate (and replace any long-acting insulin you were injecting before), and larger bolus doses before meals and snacks based mostly on carb counts of the food you are going to eat. You are still in control of the delivery of the larger doses, as you program your pump to deliver the correct dose before you eat and in response to results of blood sugar monitoring, which you still have to do. The pump itself is worn outside the body and is relatively small— ranging from about the size of a small cell phone to slightly bigger versions that hold more insulin.

If a pump is right for you, you will probably be able to find one that you like, depending on which features are important to you. However, insulin pumps are not for everyone. If you can achieve blood glucose control that you are satisfied with using multiple injections, then there may be no reason to get a pump. Although some people find it more convenient to use a pump instead of giving six to eight injections a day, having a pump is still a commitment. It is not foolproof, so you always have to have a backup insulin handy. It comes with specific challenges—namely the ones that I call the "Four S's"—style, swimming, showering, and sex. Before committing to an insulin pump, it is helpful to hear what others have to say about it. You can visit forums at www.insulinpumpforums.com or www.insulin-pumpers.org, which also has a great list of FAQs and articles about the specifics of using an insulin pump, such as where to wear your pump, traveling with your pump, and pictures of different infusion sites.

Drugs for People With Type 2 Diabetes

People with type 2 diabetes have a number of drugs that work with the insulin that their body produces to help control blood sugar, whereas people with type 1 diabetes have to get all of their insulin from the outside. Of course, many people with type 2 diabetes take some form of insulin, many in combination with some of these drugs.

Basically, each of the medications for type 2 diabetes does one or more of three things: it increases insulin production, it helps insulin (made by the body or injected) work better, and it slows down food absorption. Here is an overview of the different classes of these drugs and their mechanisms of action:

Drugs to Increase Insulin Production

Sulfonylureas. This is the oldest class of oral diabetes drugs. It works by stimulating the pancreas to produce more insulin. It is taken once or twice a day and works quickly. The main side effects are hypoglycemia, nausea, and weight gain. Sulfonylureas include glimepiride (Amaryl), glipizide (Glucotrol), glipizide ER (Glucotrol XL), and glyburide (DiaBeta, Glynase PresTab, Micronase).

Meglitinides. These drugs, also known as "glinides," increase insulin production in response to glucose circulating in the bloodstream. For this reason, they are taken 5 to 30 minutes before eating. These meds also work quickly. The main side effects are hypoglycemia and weight gain. Meglitinides include repaglinide (Prandin) and nateglinide (Starlix).

Incretin mimetics/Glucagon-like peptide (GLP)-1 Analogs. These drugs get the pancreas to make more insulin by "mimicking" the incretin hormones, which are produced in the gastrointestinal tract. They also delay the rate at which glucose enters the bloodstream by slowing digestion. In fact, some people lose weight on these medications, as they feel full for longer and eat less as a result. These drugs are injected twice a day within 60 minutes of eating. The most common side effects of these drugs are nausea, dizziness, and headaches. They can contribute to kidney problems, so they cannot be taken by anyone with diabetes-related kidney dysfunction. Incretin mimetics/GLP-1 Analogs include exenatide (Byetta) and liraglutide (Victoza).

Dipeptidyl peptidase (DPP)-4 inhibitors. These drugs lower glucose levels by keeping insulin available for the body to use longer by blocking an enzyme (DPP-4) that normally works to destroy a protein that keeps insulin in the bloodstream. Some of the advantages of these drugs are that they don't cause people to gain weight and only have to be taken orally once a day. Some of the most common side effects are respiratory infections and headaches; however, there is also an increased incidence of pancreatitis, which is much more serious. DPP-4 inhibitors include sitagliptin (Januvia) and saxagliptin (Onglyza).

Drugs to Make Insulin Work Better

Biguanides. The most commonly prescribed drugs for type 2 diabetes, these meds work by lowering glucose produced by the liver after digestion and improving glucose absorption by lowering insulin resistance. These drugs have several things going for them—they do not lead to weight gain (and may even help with weight loss). They may also lower low-density lipoprotein (LDL) cholesterol and triglyceride levels. These drugs should be taken with extreme caution (or not at all) by people with kidney problems or heart failure, as these people are at greater risk for potentially fatal accumulation of lactic acid in the bloodstream called lactic acidosis. Biguanides include metformin (Glucophage, Glucophage XR), glipizide and metformin (Metaglip), metformin and glyburide (Glucovance), repaglinide and metformin (Prandimet), and rosiglitazone and metformin (Avandamet).

Thiazolidinediones. These drugs, commonly known as TZDs, lower blood glucose levels by making fat and muscle cells more receptive to insulin. Although these drugs may help raise high-density lipoprotein (HDL) cholesterol and only need to be taken once or twice a day, they also have some distinct disadvantages. Avandia now carries a black box warning of an increased risk of fatal heart attacks on this drug after a study showed that people taking Avandia were 43% more likely to have a heart attack than people on other diabetes drugs. In fact, *Consumer Reports Best Buy Drugs report on Treating Type 2 Diabetes: The Oral Diabetes Drugs* states:

> Don't Take Avandia . . . While more research is needed to verify the magnitude of the risk posed by Avandia—and whether it should remain available—we join other groups (including the

American Diabetes Association, American Heart Association, and the American College of Cardiology) in urging you to talk to your doctor about the appropriateness of this choice. If your doctor prescribes Avandia as the first diabetes drug you take after diagnosis, you should question that decision.

In addition to this extreme (and rare) side effect, these drugs can also cause weight gain, raise levels of LDL cholesterol, and may cause liver problems. Thiazolidinediones include rosiglitazone (Avandia), pioglitazone (Actos), and rosiglitazone and metformin (Avandamet).

Drugs to Slow Down Food Absorption

Alpha-glucosidase inhibitors. These drugs are taken before each meal to slow digestion by blocking or delaying starch from being absorbed by the intestines, which slows glucose production. Usually, these medications are taken in combination with other drugs. They have the additional plus of not causing weight gain and the side effect profile here is pretty benign, with the most common effects reported being nausea, diarrhea, or gas. Alpha-glucosidase inhibitors include miglitol (Glyset) and acarbose (Precose).

Anti-hyperglycemic/synthetic form of amylin. Pramlintide (Symlin) is a newer drug, which is an artificial form of a hormone called amylin. It works to delay the emptying of the contents of the stomach, which in turn slows the release of glucose from the liver. This results in reduced absorption of carbohydrates, meaning that blood glucose levels are lower after meals. This drug must be injected. It is used in combination with insulin by both people with type 1 diabetes and people with type 2 diabetes, injected 15 minutes before meals. This drug has the benefit of helping people lose weight by making them feel "full" for much longer after eating. It can increase the risk of severe hypoglycemia, so people need to be very careful when taking it, and they should have strategies in place to lessen its risk and should promptly address any hypoglycemia.

A Note About Insulin for People With Type 2 Diabetes

For many people with type 2 diabetes, insulin is an emotionally charged topic. It may start with an inexperienced (or just crappy) doctor threatening a newly diagnosed person with "the needle" if he or she doesn't exercise and diet his or her way out of insulin resistance. Many people remember Uncle Don injecting himself with insulin until the day that he died from kidney failure, leading many people to erroneously make the causal association between insulin use and bad outcomes. In fact, in one study, 35% of participants believed that insulin actually causes blindness, amputations, heart attacks, strokes, and renal failure.[1]

For some people, insulin represents failure and corresponding shame, as it is interpreted by them as a sign that they have not taken care of themselves. Most people in the same study mentioned earlier refused to start insulin because they "planned to change health behaviors."

It is estimated that about one-third of people with type 2 diabetes for whom insulin is prescribed never refill their prescription after the first one is written, meaning that they never started it or quit taking it soon after initiation.

Statistics say that at least 50% of people diagnosed with type 2 diabetes will eventually need insulin, as their pancreas eventually cannot make enough insulin to cover their needs, despite "help" from the oral meds to produce and use insulin.

If you are super-resistant to the idea of insulin, you may want to really think about why that is so. Many people with type 2 diabetes report that they had no idea how tired they were or how bad they felt until they started taking insulin and felt better. You may be one of those people. If your doctor recommends insulin, you may want to give it a try—not as a "last resort" and not as a sign of failure, but as a better, more effective way to control blood glucose.

In fact, you may want to initiate the conversation with your doctor, as many doctors delay bringing up insulin as an option, because of the mistaken assumption that the patient cannot "handle" insulin or will not be adherent. This sort of judgment call, without discussion with the patient, leads to both the person with diabetes and the doctor tolerating poor blood glucose control unnecessarily before all options have been explored.

Aspects of Treatment to Consider

Usually the first thing we want to know about a medication is how well it works for our condition. In fact, as we sit on the exam table while the doctor is writing the prescription and telling us that this will help us control our blood sugar or treat/prevent complications better and more easily than before, we often forget to ask about anything else.

Then we get our prescription filled and notice that there are some unexpected aspects to this new med—maybe an unpleasant side effect pops up or the dosing is inconvenient—so we don't take it as often as we should. It goes without saying that even a "miracle drug" won't work if it isn't taken. Therefore, I encourage all of you to look at the following list of factors that must be weighed when making a treatment decision. Many of these are things that the doctor should know or consider in choosing what he or she thinks is right, but you should be aware of them, and mention them, as well. This list is not complete, by any means, but highlights some of the other aspects of drugs that may be deal breakers for people under certain circumstances.

Type of Diabetes

Clearly, whether you have type 1 or type 2 diabetes establishes certain parameters within which drugs are prescribed. In addition, people with latent autoimmune diabetes in adults (LADA) and a certain percentage of people with type 2 diabetes will find their choices become increasingly restricted as time after diagnosis passes as a result of their pancreas diminishing insulin production.

Ease of Glucose Control

Within each type of diabetes are people for whom glucose control is relatively easily attained and dramatic swings are rare. Other people struggle almost constantly, feeling like they are "walking a tightrope" between outrageously high glucose levels and severe hypoglycemia as they strive for control. Most people fall in the middle of these extremes. Your situation will determine what kind of medications you are on. Your situation may also change, and your meds may need to be changed as well—you may start an intensive exercise program that alters your needs, or, in another example, your body's insulin production may be lessening with time. Different classes of drugs may make glucose control more easily attainable.

Dosing Frequency

When meds are first prescribed, we often don't really know what "3 times a day" or "15 minutes before eating" means in real life, especially if we are trying to integrate new drugs into an existing regimen.

However, combine a couple of medications requiring frequent dosing or very specific timing, and it seems that there is always a forgotten pill or the undesirable situation of trying to schedule eating "after this drug, but before this other drug, allowing a minimum of 30 minutes in between, not to exceed 60 minutes." Think through your lifestyle and current list of meds before you sign on to one that may complicate matters. If you have a hectic schedule or unpredictable mealtimes, some drugs may be better choices than others.

Weight Gain

Several studies have shown that one of the main reasons that people stop taking their diabetes meds is because of the weight gain that is associated with many of these drugs. Insulin and the sulfonylureas may cause hypoglycemia, which stimulates appetite, leading to weight gain. The thiazolidinediones cause fat cells to enlarge and can also cause fluid retention, which both result in higher numbers on the scale. Regardless of the mechanism, weight gain is particularly frustrating for most people—especially people with diabetes who are overweight or obese, as "losing weight" is often one of the components in their diabetes management strategy. The average weight gain on these drugs is between 5 and 10 pounds, so not a huge amount, but it can be stressful to see the numbers on the scale moving in the wrong direction if you are trying to lose weight. (Note: There are ways to limit weight gain by working with your doctor or certified diabetes educator (CDE) to plan ahead to increase activity and change food intake—you *can* decrease the number of pounds gained and improve blood glucose if you strategize this.)

Injections vs. Pills (or Other Delivery Mechanisms)

This might not be something you have a great deal of choice about. Currently, all insulin are delivered by injection or pump, so if insulin is part of your treatment regimen, there will be some needles in your life. (It looks like a form of insulin, which is to be inhaled, is making its way to market, but even this will not replace all injected insulin for certain people.)

There are also non-insulin drugs, such as Symlin (pramlintide) and Byetta (exenatide), that are injected, and your doctor may want to put you on one of these. Byetta (exenatide) is taken by people with type 2 diabetes and may be the first injectable drug that has ever been prescribed.

Trying to Conceive

Many of the oral drugs for type 2 diabetes are contraindicated during pregnancy, so you will definitely want to mention to your doctor if you are trying to conceive, so that he or she can make sure you are on the safest treatment for yourself and your future baby, as well as work closely with you during this period to help you optimize blood glucose control. Also, regardless if you have type 1 or type 2 diabetes, you will want to go see your doctor as soon as you get pregnant to strategize your treatment, as medication and monitoring needs may change drastically throughout your pregnancy.

Contraindications

People with certain conditions cannot take certain drugs. For instance, people with kidney dysfunction or heart failure cannot take metformin, as this can lead to a dangerous condition called lactic acidosis. Byetta (exenatide) cannot be taken by people with kidney problems, as one of the common side effects is vomiting, which can lower the volume of fluid in the body and damage the kidneys.

You may think that it is your doctor's business to know which drugs are potentially dangerous to you before deciding on a medication. Although you may be right in principle, research shows that contraindicated drugs are frequently prescribed. A 2003 study showed that of 100 patients that had been prescribed metformin, 22 had at least one contraindication (kidney problems or heart failure).[2] Although it is important to have confidence in your doctor, ultimately, we are the people that are putting the medications in our bodies and should check out these drugs before we do so (see "Get A Handle on Your Treatment Options" in this chapter for tips on researching medications).

Your Doctor's Opinion

Your doctor may have a very strong opinion about which therapy he or she would like to see you on—so strong, in fact, that it leaves little room for discussion. Although I am a big advocate of not allowing myself to be bullied, I also think that there are often very good reasons why a doctor might "insist" on a certain treatment strategy—maybe he or she had patients that were very similar to you who did very well on a particular drug or combination of drugs. Your doctor could also have solid grounds for disliking a medication—he or she may have had a cluster of people experiencing the same "rare" side effect or have been forced to switch too many people off a drug that they failed to respond to. If your doctor "tells" you what medication you "will" be taking, ask your doctor why he or she feels strongly about it—the reasons may be much more convincing than yours, especially if you were wavering between a couple of treatments, and it was coming down to a decision based on a slightly higher co-pay or a dosing schedule that was a little more inconvenient. However, it is still important that you understand why your doctor is so adamantly recommending this treatment.

Take Charge

Don't forget to ask your doctor "why?" when he or she makes a therapy recommendation. Your doctor's "why" response should be thoughtful and make sense to you.

On the other hand, your doctor may say that your treatment decision is entirely up to you (within certain limits, of course). In this case, it still doesn't hurt to ask your doctor what he or she thinks would be the best course for you. I often use the approach of asking, "If I was your sister, what would you recommend and why?" Some doctors might not like that question, but it usually elicits an honest opinion.

Take Charge

Don't expect your doctor's office to call to remind you to schedule your next appointment. At the end of every visit or treatment, be sure to ask when the next treatment or follow-up visit should be. Don't leave your doctor's office or the treatment center without having scheduled that appointment (or at least noting the time frame in your calendar).

Cost

Your treatment decision may be easier if your insurance covers one drug with a co-pay of $10 per month versus another drug that is not covered and would cost $300 each month. At that point, for many of us, the decision is made. You may also be in a situation where one manufacturer may have a patient assistance program that you qualify for and the others don't.

Sticker Shock?

I am pretty sure that nobody likes to have to spend money on medications, people with diabetes included. In fact, several studies have shown that cost is a big factor in whether people are going to take their diabetes meds at all (especially if they don't understand why they need the drugs or how they work). In one study, for every 10-dollar increase in monthly co-pay for their medications, there was a 26% increase in the likelihood that people would stop taking their meds altogether (67% of people who had a co-pay of $30 or more discontinued therapy in the first year).[3] Another study of people on oral antidiabetic medications showed that every 5-dollar increase in monthly co-pay for drugs corresponded to a 0.1% increase in A1c results.[4]

The world of chronic disease is a big eye-opener when it comes to drug prices. It would be shocking enough to grapple with the idea of paying hundreds of dollars for a month's worth of meds, but then we have to get our heads around the fact that this is not just for 1 month— oh no, those calendar pages keep flipping and we are talking about lots of money for a long time.

It is helpful to have health insurance, but drugs still might cost quite a bit, because of things like complications with formularies or choice of specialty pharmacies, which may mean that we find ourselves paying substantial percentages of drug costs, rather than a fixed co-pay amount. If you have health insurance, the first thing to do is to line up your prescription meds and call your insurance company and see if there is any way to reduce the money that you are paying out of pocket. You might also take a look and see if you are getting generics, which can make a huge difference for some of the drugs.

DestinationRx (**www.destinationrx.com**) is a helpful site, which allows you to compare prices on drugs, check out generic options, and manage your list of medications. Just to see what it was all about, I searched "glucophage" to see what the price differences were and had the following information on prices per month of medication returned: "The least amount your drug costs: $60.59. The maximum amount your drug costs: $69.99." When I clicked on the "Comparable Drug" tab, a generic option popped up for metformin hcl for $4.00. Seems like it may be worth a conversation with your doctor to see if he or she is comfortable with a generic in this case.

Prescription drug cards may help ease the pain a little. Two to check out are *RxDrugCard* (**www.rxdrugcard.com**) or 888-216-2461, through which members pay a small yearly fee to receive discounts at participating pharmacies; or *Together Rx Access Card* (**www.togetherrxaccess.com**) or 800-444-4106, which is free, but limited to people who have no prescription drug coverage and meet certain income guidelines.

Patient assistance programs exist for many of the drugs used to treat diabetes, as well as for many of the glucose monitoring supplies, like meters and strips. You can check with the manufacturer or you can look at some of the Web sites that have organized much of the information about the various programs in one place in easy-to-search formats, which can help you figure out eligibility and provide application forms for different programs. My favorite ones, for ease of searching and comprehensiveness, are *NeedyMeds* (**www.needymeds.com**) and *The Partnership for Prescription Assistance* (**www.pparx.org**).

Get a Handle on Your Treatment Options

Figuring out what medical options are available to you can be a challenging task. There may be other drugs that could give your relief from your complications or help you keep your glucose more stable. Your current drug regimen might not be the best for you. It may seem that you have exhausted your options, but there just might be something else out there.

Many people would say that it is up to your doctor to figure all of this out and that looking at other options is a waste of a patient's time. Bah, I say. Although there may be things that are clearly wrong for you, there may be things that your doctor hasn't necessarily thought of for your particular case. There may be doctors who are trying different approaches with great success on cases like yours, even if your doctor says there is nothing else to be done. It is not about challenging your doctor in a negative or angry way, it is about looking at all of your options. There is a good chance that your doctor will try something new, refer you to someone who is using that therapy on his or her patients, or at least look into it more if you ask.

It helps to have a system to weed out the false options, to figure out what meds might work well together and make a decision about your approach. I will present some ideas on how to tackle this exploration of what is out there. You will gather some information about the options that are available to you. Then you'll do an analysis of each one. By the end of the exercise, you will have a fairly complete list of possibilities, along with your notes and the opinions of some trusted sources. This can be used now or in the future to guide your decision-making process.

First, discuss your options with your doctor. He or she may have very strong opinions about what you should be on. This may be based on experiences with patients fitting a similar profile as you or may be just a personal preference to start everyone on a certain drug. If your doctor says something along the lines of, "We are starting you on Glucophage XR next week," your discussion (and decision making) may be over. You may also have a condition that limits your treatment options. However, I recommend that you still do the research discussed later to see what you are getting into and to make sure that you are comfortable with the treatment plan. Do not hesitate to make another appointment or call your doctor on the phone if you have questions or want to discuss other options.

I suspect most doctors fall into the "middle ground," setting parameters from within that you can choose, or suggesting that you give something a try for a couple of months to see how it works for you. Many doctors will say, "In my opinion. . ." but then listen when you present your side, especially if you have specific concerns. Usually, you can end up with a compromise—to try it your way or the doctor's way for a little while, agreeing to reassess the situation in the future.

Start by creating your form. On a piece of paper make the following columns: "Medication," "What It Is For" (if it is a disease-modifying therapy or for a specific symptom), "Risks/Side Effects," "Benefits," "Cost," and "Miscellaneous." Fill in the columns as you conduct your search.

Look online. I think the first place to start the search is online, if you are comfortable with the Internet. I recommend a two-stage approach to researching these drugs. First, gather the objective facts. Go on *MedlinePlus* (**www.medlineplus.gov**) or the *American Diabetes Association* (**www.diabetes.org**) Web site to learn the basics of the meds, such as how often you will need to take them, anticipated side effects, and efficacy. If you want to look deeper into these drugs at this point, go through the exercises in the next section, "Learn More About Your Meds" to conduct an even more in-depth research.

The Real World

There's a lot of crappy nonsense online about diabetes. Stick to reliable sources until you are confident that you can separate nonsense from valuable information.

For my second (and probably most important) step in my Internet research, I would recommend finding out what "the people" have to say. There are plenty of places to find out about the experiences of people who have tried these drugs. Here are a couple of my favorites:

Revolution Health. Found at **www.revolutionhealth.com/drugs-treatments**, this resource used to be called "RemedyFind." It allows actual people who are using different medications to write in and rate a drug in four areas (perceived effectiveness, tolerability, ease of use, would you recommend?) as well as write in an entry on the drug. Visit it and read what people have to say—it is fascinating. Again, remember that people who have very positive or very negative experiences are more likely to take the time to write to such a site, but the entries still provide pretty interesting perspectives. To get to the relevant part, click on "Drugs and Treatments" in the top menu bar, then enter the name of your drug of interest in the search bar. Click on "Read all [drug name] ratings" under the "user ratings" column when it comes up. Play around on the site—there are ways to limit searches to your type of diabetes or complication.

Do Your Best

People online can be strange or have completely different ideas from you, but the more opinions you read, the more you will understand. Get stories from more than one place and actively seek out differing points of view.

Ask A Patient database. You can find this one at **www.askapatient.com**. Also informative, this site focuses entirely on patient feedback about drugs. Askapatient.com has a more "homemade" feel than the Revolution Health site (but seems to be a much more popular place for people with diabetes to rate their experience with medications), mostly focusing on side effects, although people are asked to submit an overall rating for the drug. An interesting feature of this site is that some people provide e-mail addresses in case you want to ask a question directly.

DailyStrength. Go to **www.dailystrength.org**. This is also a patient-rating site, where people can say if a drug is "working" or "not working." People only post a tiny bit of information on each drug (sample entries for Metformin include "a real gut killer" and "helps with my weight loss—everything goes straight out of me"). Some neat features of DailyStrength are that you can send a message to each person and most people have all of the drugs that they are taking posted under their profiles with comments. The site is a little confusing and requires a little "messing around" on it to get the hang of what is happening. However, there are pretty interesting discussions going on in the forums.

Take Charge
Value others' opinions, but form your own.

Ask a pharmacist. This is a profession that people do not fully use, as many have the impression of the pharmacists in our local stores as being mere "pill counters." A PharmD (Doctor of Pharmacy) in a drugstore can be an invaluable source of information and often have much more time than doctors to explain medications. Talk to your pharmacist about any medications you are on, side effects, and potential interactions and tap into the pharmacist's wealth of knowledge about the stuff we put into our bodies.

Talk to people. Of course, this is a good thing to do if you have the opportunity. However, if you are in a support group, you can ask for input, opinions, and experiences around medications. Prepare yourself for a long session, as people usually love to talk about their medication experiences. Also, keep in mind that some people are very adamant about their choices, so you may be asked about your decision (and find yourself in the position of defending it if your final choice differed from their advice).

Evaluate. We all have different things that we are looking for, or trying to avoid, when choosing a treatment. If your insurance doesn't cover a certain drug, don't bother looking at it any further, unless there are other options for paying for it. There is no point in comparing statistical data on specific drugs if there is an insurmountable barrier to taking some of them. The final choice will be a combination of many factors, including your lifestyle and your doctor endorsing your treatment plan.

Now, repeat step #1 and talk to your doctor. Tell your doctor your ideas around medications. Tell him or her the main reasons for your choices—be specific. However, be prepared to compromise if your doctor has valid reasons for suggesting a different treatment strategy.

The Real World
Make sure that it is you who makes decisions, not your fears, your diabetes, your friends, or your procrastination. Make your decisions yourself and be proud of them.

Learn More About Your Meds

There are many examples of possible—even probable—drug interactions that could occur for a person with diabetes. People with diabetes often end up taking a cornucopia of meds: From our endocrinologist we will get medications for managing our blood glucose. We may have a couple things thrown into the mix to handle associated problems, like high cholesterol or high blood pressure. I know I don't hesitate to run out and purchase entire drugstore aisles of over-the-counter medications when I have a hint of an allergy or a cold. Then, there are the vitamins and supplements that seem innocuous. Many women also take contraceptives to prevent unplanned pregnancies or hormone replacement therapy after menopause. All of these things can interact with each other and with your diabetes.

Do Your Best

Every medication, even over-the-counter vitamin supplements and remedies, should be carefully tracked for interactions and side effects. Read the labels, search online, and ask each one of your health providers about your meds.

Given the various stuff that may be going into our bodies, it is pretty unlikely that any of your doctors are aware of all of the medications or supplements that you are using. Even if they are, it is very difficult for them to keep up with all of the potential interactions that may occur. You cannot rely on the pharmacists' computer alert programs to track it all, either, as we may get some of our medications from different pharmacies or by mail order. In addition, our pharmacists have no way of knowing what types of supplements and over-the-counter stuff we are taking.

Therefore, it is up to you to do some research on the drugs that you are taking or considering taking. I recommend making a little list or chart with the following columns: "Medication/Dosage," "Interactions," "Misc./Special Instructions," "Side Effects," and "Doctor Notes." In the "Medication" column, list the medications you are taking and the dosages. I would include any over-the-counter things you are taking and supplements that are beyond a daily multivitamin (like St. John's wort or SAM-e).

The "Interactions" column is simple. List those drugs that you are currently taking or considering taking. You can also list things that may come up later, like certain kinds of antidepressants or medications to treat complications, if these are symptoms that you have that may require medication in the future.

The "Misc./Special Instructions" column holds things that you didn't know about your med, but you discover during your research.

These may be instructions that help reduce side effects or increase the effectiveness of the drug, and may include things like "don't drink grapefruit juice while using this medication" or "take at the same time every day." Also, include any contraindications that apply to you specifically, such as "not recommended for people with high blood pressure" or "should not be used by people with kidney dysfunction."

"Side Effects" is where you list those things that you may be experiencing, but didn't know that they were related to any drug until you saw it listed as part of a description of a medication that you are taking. This is also where you make a special note of those potential side effects that are mentioned in conjunction with a warning to "call your doctor immediately if you experience any of these symptoms."

The "Doctor Notes" column is your space to note what you want to mention to your physician and what questions you may have. It is also a place where you can record what his or her answer was.

The following are the online places that I recommend for starting your research. Although it may seem like overkill, I really believe that you should look at more than one place (at the very least MedlinePlus and PDR Health):

MedlinePlus (www.medlineplus.gov). Again, I really love MedlinePlus, which is a service provided by the US government (the National Library of Medicine and the National Institutes of Health). This site tends to include much more detailed information than I have seen anywhere else. However, you have to read each entry pretty carefully, as the authors have lumped information about interactions, contraindications, and special instructions together under the heading of "What Special Precautions Should I Follow?" Still, this is the place to start.

PDR Health (www.pdrhealth.com). This is the consumer site maintained by the publishers of *Physician's Desk Reference* (the main drug resource that doctors use—it's the big red book that is sitting on their desk or in their Palm Pilot), so it is probably the most up-to-date. This site has nice detailed information about how the drug should be taken, for instance, what you should do if you miss a dose, and if it should be taken with food (also mentioning if food will delay its effects).

Know Your Stuff

When researching treatments (or anything else), look up words you don't know. In Google, just type *define:[search term]* for a list of definitions.

Drug Interactions Checker. A service on the Drugs.com site **(www .drugs.com)**, this is an incredibly easy way to figure out if all your medications are going to play nicely with each other. All you do is enter the names of all the drugs you are on, including herbals, vitamin and mineral supplements, and over-the-counter medications. Then, click the "Check Interactions" button, and you've got yourself information that would have taken hours to track down any other way. One thing that I *highly recommend* doing—the Drug Interactions Checker also allows you to see what kind of harm you can do to yourself by combining caffeine, alcohol, and all sorts of illicit drugs (the database lists heroin, methamphetamine, hashish, and cocaine, among others) with each other, as well as with prescription meds and over-the-counter stuff. If you are going to be using these things, DO this research. It could literally save your life.

Do Your Best

If you dabble in illicit drugs or drink a little (or a lot of) alcohol, that is your business (mostly). However, it is also your business to make sure that these things are not interacting with your medications in a harmful way. Don't be stupid.

Besides finding out which drugs and supplements interact with each other, to what degree they interact, what the mechanism is, and what kind of problems the interactions might cause, you will also learn which meds are affected by taking them too soon after eating. By registering on the site, you are able to save your medications list, so that you can easily change it or check out drugs that you are considering in the future without having to reenter the whole thing. You can also print out the results of your research to show to your doctor. Yep, it is clear that a smart group of people were using their heads (and testing how real people would use the Drug Interaction function) when they put this site together. The rest of the site is pretty spectacular, as well.

Manufacturer's site. I also like going to the manufacturer's Web site for the prescribing information available to physicians. Usually, typing the drug name into your search engine, such as Google or Yahoo, will get you to the site right away—most brand-name medications have their own site. This is where you are most likely to see any serious warnings first. By looking at the "Full Prescribing Information," you are seeing everything the drug company wants the doctor to know while avoiding language and images designed to convince you that you need this drug.

Some people may find the full version of the prescribing information a bit overwhelming. Most companies now provide a "Patient Information" sheet that contains much of the same information in a more easily understood format with less medical terminology.

Now what? First of all, don't overreact to any of the information you have found. Of course, take action right away if you have one of those "contact your doctor immediately" side effects. However, if you find out that your allergy medicine may reduce the effect of a certain drug, there is no need to freak out. You do need to ask your doctor about it as soon as possible, though. Look over your list and compile all the questions that you have. If there are some questions that require an immediate answer, call your doctor's office. Otherwise, you may have to make an appointment to get all of your questions answered.

Monitor Effects (and Side Effects) of Medications

Many people with type 2 diabetes feel "just fine" before they are diagnosed. All of a sudden, they are then asked to take drugs required to "keep them healthy" that may actually make them feel worse initially than they did before diagnosis, although many of these side effects usually disappear or become more tolerable as time passes. In addition, diabetes doctors may prescribe statins, beta-blockers, ACE inhibitors, and other medications to help reduce risk of complications, which make some people feel tired, weak, dizzy, or just less good than they would like. Keeping a medication effects log can help guide decisions around medications and help doctors optimize treatment, while possibly reducing side effects.

Make It Better

The symptoms of diabetes, its complications, side effects of diabetes medications, and treatment for complications all overlap and interact to make a big complicated mess. Take control by paying attention to all the factors that make you feel better or worse.

Keep a Medication Effects Log

It is extremely important for us to monitor the effects of the medications that we take for our diabetes and any complications we might have to make sure that we are getting the most out of them and that they are the right meds for us. In the case of many of our symptoms and complications, the doctors rely on our reports of improvement (or not) to decide if or how to continue treatment with these drugs, so it is crucial that we be accurate and provide our doctor with good-quality information.

Take Charge

Do you know all the potential side effects of each of your medications? Maybe something you had been blaming on diabetes is really a side effect. A simple medication modification from your doctor could lessen some of your symptoms. Discuss any suspected side effects with your doctor or pharmacist.

In addition, side effects of medications can often be lessened by changing simple things, like time of day the drugs are taken or splitting doses. It is also possible that what you think might be the beginnings of a new complication are side effects of medication, and vice versa. Logging can help prevent unnecessary suffering and stress.

Using a simple form that you make, you will periodically record when you take your medications, your symptom intensity and duration, as well as note any other factors that may be affecting your symptoms.

Make a list. Write the date at the top of the paper, you'll use at least one sheet per day. Next, draw six columns on the paper—the first four columns should be narrow and the last column wider. The columns should be labeled "Time," "Medication," "Effect," "Severity," "Blood Glucose," and "Other Factors." In the "Time" column, fill in the hours that you are awake, 1 hour per line (7:00 AM, 8:00 AM, and so on). In the "Medication" column, you will write down the medication you take next to the corresponding time. In the "Effect" column, write down anything that you notice that seems related to the medication, next to the corresponding time or noting the time. In the "Severity" column, you'll write how severe the symptom is on a scale of 1 to 10 ("10" being the worst you could imagine). In the "Other Factors" column, you'll note food you have eaten, activities or exercise that you have engaged in, your stress level, or anything else that might influence the symptom. Here's an example of an entry—Time: 7:15 PM (right before dinner); Medication: Glucophage 500 mg; Effect: 10:25 PM, diarrhea; Severity: 6; Blood Glucose: 142 at 10:40 PM; Other Factors: did not eat much dinner. Keep in mind that you may not fill in every field every time that you make an entry.

Keep it with you. If you have your medication effects log with you, it will be much easier to make entries. Don't rely on your memory at the end of the day. Jot notes on an index card during the day and enter them on the form each evening if it is easier.

Make entries. Stop at least four times during the day to check in and make entries. The more often you stop and enter observations, the more accurate your medication effects log will be. This is especially important if you are trying to figure out what triggers or helps specific things or side effects. Set a timer or alarm to remind yourself to check in with your symptoms, stress, or energy levels. Try to be as detailed and specific as possible. It will make it easier to see patterns later.

List other factors. Although the main columns on your medication effects log are self-explanatory, the "Other Factors" column could be the most important. Here is where you will try to capture and note other things that may influence how you feel. Besides just the medication that you are taking, social situations, food, your mood, and the temperature outside may all influence how you experience a symptom. Be sure to note these things.

Take Charge

Become your own medical detective and ruthlessly analyze every change in how you feel.

Analyze. Analyze your data every couple of days. This will help you to see patterns in the items you are tracking, as well as improve your data input. Look for patterns in the time of day, the duration and severity of symptoms, as well as any potential side effect (or positive effects) from the medications. Take a good look at the other factors and see if you can identify things that make symptoms worse, as well as things that may help.

Make some changes (after discussing with your doctor). While still keeping your medication effects log, make some changes. You may want to take the drug a little closer to mealtime or adjust your whole schedule of eating and medication by an hour or two to space your doses a little further apart. However, all these things must be mentioned to your doctor or checked with the nurse to ensure that (1) the effects that you are noticing are not an indication of a serious adverse reaction, and (2) that it is okay to take the meds with more or less food, closer to eating, further apart, etc. If the medication makes you dizzy for an hour, make sure that you strategically time your morning showers, driving a car, or anything else that could put you (or others) in danger.

To go more in-depth with your medication effects log, try logging everything for a week. In addition to any symptoms you might have, log moods, sleep, energy level, stress level, and productivity. By logging everything, you can really start to see connections between your behaviors and how you feel. This could give you new ideas about how to improve your health.

Don't forget to log contact with people. Some people can literally cause you pain and stress, although others may lift your mood and help you forget about your symptoms.

With pain or other chronic symptoms, note if there are times during the day when you are not as bothered by them—what is happening during those times? You can use your log to identify both negative and positive factors.

Help Your Meds Help You

Okay, so you have the drugs in your hands (or in your fridge or medicine cabinet), but just can't get around to getting the medicine into your body, or end up taking them on a random schedule. Not only does this (greatly) lower the possibility that the drugs can help you, but this lack of adherence also causes all sorts of guilt and stress that is unnecessary. Remember, in this book, we are focusing on taking control of our situation, so if you have decided to be on a medication to help control your glucose or treat a complication, let's get this fixed. The following are some "barriers to adherence" and ideas to overcome them. Often, just recognizing them in yourself and acknowledging them has a great effect on helping you get past these problems.

Know Your Stuff

Adherence means that you take your medication *exactly* as prescribed, without skipping doses or allowing too much time to lapse between doses.

Do Your Best

Medications don't work if you don't take them correctly. Missed doses and not following instructions just create more confusion in trying to find the right treatment strategy for you. Take your medicine, and take it correctly.

People With Type 2 Diabetes Unwilling to Take Insulin

Although many people with type 2 diabetes will eventually need to take insulin to control their blood sugar, about a third of these people are so reluctant to do so that they refuse to start or quit shortly after beginning therapy. Some of the reasons for this resistance to the whole idea of insulin are common to other diabetes drugs (discussed later), such as dislike or phobia of needles and weight gain. However, insulin also carries with it unique negative associations for many people. The need for insulin makes many people feel guilty or like they have failed at managing their diabetes. Often, people feel like they have now "crossed a line" with their diabetes—that it is now a serious condition that will require constant monitoring and inconvenient or complicated dosing. They may associate insulin with loved ones who had complications or did not take care of themselves. People may be scared of hypoglycemic "episodes" or otherwise causing themselves harm from not administering the insulin correctly.

Pro-adherence Strategy

Share decision making with the doctor. A big part of the problem with adherence in many cases is that the patients are passive, waiting for the doctor to "tell them what to do." Many of these people smile and nod while the doctor is laying out the strategy and accept the prescription that the doctor holds out to them, although knowing that they are not going to get it filled. On the other hand, they may truly believe that they are going to follow through, but decide later that they can handle the situation better themselves through diet and exercise. In the case of insulin, there needs to be buy-in for the treatment to work—after all, you have to do things that you think may be unpleasant and/or inconvenient, like monitor your blood glucose more frequently and inject yourself. It is important that you share your concerns with your doctor. Tell him or her if you absolutely do not want to start insulin or set up some conditions under which you will give it a try. Let your doctor explain his or her thinking around starting insulin and address your concerns. You may just find yourself agreeing with the strategy when you understand the rationale behind it better and goals that the doctor has in mind for your glucose control.

Counseling and Education

Maybe you are willing to give it a go and try insulin. However, you think it's complicated. Like most people, you have never given yourself an injection and are not sure you are doing it right. Or, you have an overseas trip planned and have absolutely no idea what to do with your insulin when you are traveling, not knowing if you can bring syringes on airplanes, or how you can stay on your injection schedule when there is a 9-hour time difference at your destination. A CDE can answer all of these questions and any other concern you may have. Ask your doctor for a referral. In fact, ask your doctor for a referral to a CDE before you start insulin, so that you can discuss your concerns before they cause you stress in real life.

Fear of Weight Gain

Yes, it is unfair that one of the "cornerstones" of treatment of diabetes is weight loss and weight control, yet several of the medications (including insulin) in the diabetes medicine chest make this difficult and may even cause weight gain. Studies show that this fear of gaining weight is a huge barrier to adherence, enough so that many people simply refuse to take these drugs.[5-7] Insulin does this by helping the body use glucose more efficiently and reducing the body's metabolic rate, which means that the same number of calories are turned into fat more easily than before the insulin was introduced.

Pro-adherence Strategy

I don't know if this comes as good news or bad news to you, but the formula to avoiding weight gain with insulin is pretty much the same old stuff: weight control = reducing calories + increasing activity. This is a great topic to discuss with your CDE.

Check into other medications. For some people (especially those with type 2 diabetes), there are medications that can be combined with insulin to help you reduce your dosage. Some of these, including metformin, Byetta (exenatide), and Symlin (pramlintide), may actually promote weight loss. They may also help you reduce your insulin dosage.

Depression and Diabetes Fatalism[8,9]

Research shows that depression negatively affects almost every area of health. In people with diabetes, depression results in people not taking their meds. Diabetes fatalism, the belief that everything is predetermined and inevitable and nothing we do can change the course of our disease, is often linked to depression and to non-adherence.

Pro-adherence Strategy

Take a look at your emotional health. According to the *Diagnostic and Statistical Manual of Mental Disorders, Fourth Edition (DSM-IV)*, the diagnostic manual of the American Psychiatric Association, which contains the criteria used by mental health professionals to diagnose patients, you are clinically depressed if you meet the following criteria:

You have had an episode of depression lasting at least 2 weeks with at least five of the following symptoms representing a change in function: sadness, loss of interest in things you previously liked to do, change in appetite, sleeping problems, moving faster or slower than usual (that people notice), fatigue, feelings of guilt, cognitive problems, or suicidal thoughts. In addition, to be officially diagnosed with depression, the symptoms must be severe enough to upset your daily routine, seriously impair your work, or interfere with your relationships and is not just a normal reaction to the death of a loved one.

Whether you meet all of the necessary criteria for depression outlined earlier or if you think some of them are just part of having depression, it doesn't matter in terms of what you need to do next. If you feel very sad or have no interest in things around you, you absolutely need to seek help as soon as possible. Leave the diagnosis and treatment to a professional. All of us living with diabetes have more than enough to deal with and depression can affect the course of our illness, because it can affect how well or poorly we take care of ourselves.

I don't like needles at all. Humans, for the most part, are hardwired to avoid causing themselves pain. It doesn't matter how "itty-bitty, teeny-tiny, or microscopic" the needle is, the first time that many of us get a syringe or an injection pen in our hands, the first thought might be, "I can NEVER do this." Various caring and loving individuals surrounding us and hectoring us doesn't help, either. It's scary, weird, and just not natural. However, it is what it is. Currently, we only have injectable insulin and if we need it, we really have no choice but to give ourselves shots (or have someone do it for us at the beginning).

The Real World

Don't mess with your meds. Yes, the side effects can be terrible and the dosing schedule inconvenient. Commit to taking them anyway, if this is what you decided to do.

Pro-adherence Strategy

There are several things you can do to get yourself to the point that you can inject yourself. Not all of these approaches will work for everyone, and you may be someone that continues to have a hard time with injecting for a while (although most people forget why they were so afraid after just a couple of injections). Anyway, if you are fearful of injecting at this moment in time, these tips are worth a try.

- There are all sorts of things you can do to "get in the mood" for an injection, such as creative visualization, deep breathing exercises, or creating a ritual around injecting (such as preinjection music and little postinjection rewards of your choosing). One of the most effective things to do to convince yourself to inject may be to look at the clock and say, "It's 7:58. If I inject *right now*, no matter how bad it is, the whole ordeal will be over by 8:00 at the latest."

- Succeed a couple of times. I know that this one is easier said than done, but I think it is the most important aspect of successful injecting. Once you do it a couple of times, you will have the confidence to know that you can keep doing it (and the evidence that nothing terrible will happen).

I keep forgetting to take my medications. Isn't it interesting that most of us do not forget things like massage appointments, that there is chocolate cake for dessert, or that we don't have to work because it is Saturday? However, here we are with something we do (or are supposed to do) daily—take our medications—and we find ourselves forgetting to do it at least a couple of times a month.

Do Your Best

Spend 1 week focused on achieving perfect adherence. By the last day, it will be a habit.

Pro-adherence Strategy

Research has shown that you are much more likely to be adherent to your treatment if you believe in it and really think that it is working. Maybe it would help to think about the fact that your A1c result was lower at your last visit or how much more energy you have since starting insulin.

If it is truly a matter of the whole thing slipping your mind, you can put into place a number of little "reminders." Of course, there is the always-mentioned sticky note solution, or you can set an alarm to go off on your cell phone. Some people are big fans of putting their medicine bottles in places where they cannot possibly be overlooked, such as blocking access to the coffee cups.

The Bottom Line

We all know people who are extremely careful about what they eat — only choosing organic fruits and vegetables, performing advanced math to ensure that their carbohydrate to protein ratio is exactly right, and not eating food that was produced in factories that ever used trans fats—yet many of these people take whichever drug is prescribed by their doctors or that they find in the drugstore aisles, no questions asked. On the other hand are the people who smoke a pack and a half of cigarettes each day and wash down their Big Macs with a six-pack of beer, yet refuse to take medication because they don't like to put "that stuff" into their bodies. Then, there are the people who carefully think through their treatment plans, research their options, discuss them with their doctors, and end up with a bunch of medications that they then only take sporadically or not at all.

In the interest of not being overly judgmental, I will refrain from judging the people that fall into the preceding categories (at least in print here). However, I will say that influencing our body's chemistry by putting drugs into it is a pretty serious deal, to be taken, well, seriously. I will also say that not taking advantage of medications that could help us, based on reasons that we haven't even thought through, is also kind of a shame.

We are the stewards of our bodies. For better or for worse, they are a means to the end—if we want to do or be something, our bodies have to be willing and able. You might feel like your body has betrayed you by "getting" diabetes, and it might be hard to work up enthusiasm for putting in so much effort just to maintain "status quo" with your health.

In addition, unlike certain problems, like simple bacterial infections that can be cured with antibiotics, diabetes treatment comes with no guarantee, must be taken for a lifetime (in most cases), and is imperfect, often requiring constant tweaking of dosages and timing to get the optimal effect. However, it's the best we have at the moment.

Frustrating as it may be, we have to use the tools at hand to do what we can to simulate what our body is no longer doing for us—efficiently using glucose for energy. I get pissed, I hate the fact that despite my seemingly constant attempts to keep my blood glucose within a certain range that it often defies me and plummets downward or is elevated. However, I have to do this. I have to keep trying. These tools, including these medications, are what we have and we must control the parts of diabetes that we can. I also have to say that although we have much further to go in perfecting the treatment of diabetes, the advances that I have seen in my lifetime have lead to marked improvement in my quality of life—and, ultimately, that is what matters to me.

6

Create Health in New Places

As we go through our days with diabetes, the disease is never far from our thoughts as we try to estimate carbs in meals and time medication doses just right. It is normal that any new sensation that we feel gets assigned to diabetes. Don't get me wrong, diabetes is often (even usually) to blame, but sometimes we just get regular illnesses like regular people.

For instance, if I have a headache, I immediately check my blood glucose, puzzled when it is in the normal range. I do this with big stuff, too. Because I have gastroparesis and associated gastroesophageal reflux disease (GERD), I questioned my doctor when an endoscopy showed that I had Barrett's esophagus, a condition in which the cells of the lower esophagus are replaced with abnormal cells. In this case, and several others, it was a really good thing that I have a doctor that is smarter than me about medical issues and stood by his diagnosis, which had nothing to do with diabetes in my case.

Not only is it understandable to immediately perform a diabetes "inventory" (including blood glucose levels or status of certain complications) when asked about health or how we are feeling, it is human nature to focus on physical status and stop there.

However, it is a shame to think in such a diabetes-centric way, especially because the "official" definition of health is "a state of complete physical, mental, and social well-being and not merely the absence of disease or infirmity." This is the definition used by the World Health Organization since 1948.

Do Your Best

Just as you are more than your diabetes, your health is more than your diabetes or any complications that you have. Don't neglect your overall health by getting lost in your diabetes.

Don't feel bad if, like me, you focus on your diabetes, or any immediate discomfort you may have, when thinking about your health. Most people do not think about their health until something is physically wrong; health is something they either have or do not have. However, when you really think about it, this understanding of health doesn't work for all, or even most, circumstances. Imagine a young person who is physically healthy—strong, in great shape—but suffers from depression. Then consider someone with a debilitating illness, who has a rich spiritual life and enjoys a strong social support network, interacting with loved ones, and takes time to appreciate fine food, literature, and music. Who is healthier? Who "feels" better?

It is often shocking to me when I go to the doctor to find out that I have a nondiabetes problem that needs attention, as that seems a little unfair, given all the diabetes stuff I have to juggle. Fair or not, it is true that people with diabetes are subject to the same health problems as the rest of the world as a result of aging or lifestyle choices. However, we also have some of the same opportunities to increase our health, as well.

Humans are complex creatures, and there is far more to overall health than physical functioning. Granted, when we don't feel good physically, it is hard to feel "healthy." However, by putting effort into examining other aspects of health, including social health, spiritual health, and mental health, it is easier not only to put physical ailments into perspective, but also to make changes to habits that could help us feel better in general. Illnesses may change priorities and strengthen relationships. True health encompasses our bodies, our emotions, our minds, our relationships, our homes, our behaviors, and our spiritual selves. Each day you can make gains, even if you continue to have diabetes challenges

Let's take a look at some other aspects of health beyond our diabetes:

Physical health. Clearly, when we feel bad, it is hard to feel "healthy," period. However, as mentioned (and as will be discussed in the second half of this chapter), physical health is more than diabetes and its complications. It's also true that if there is something you can do to improve your physical well-being, that you will probably feel better overall, including a reduction in your diabetes-related problems.

Just think of all the things that you could do today to feel better. You could exercise, add one serving of vegetables to your lunch or dinner; or have your last cup of coffee before 3 PM, so that you can go to bed 45 minutes earlier; anything to make incremental changes to your well-being.

Emotional health. The emotional aspect of health, whether a person is living with diabetes or not, is often overlooked until constant stress manifests itself as a physical problem—headaches, gastrointestinal problems, and (yes) many diabetes symptoms can be made much worse by neglecting emotional health. Emotional health seems like such a vague term that it is difficult to sum it up in a simple definition. It is not about being happy all the time and doesn't mean that you are grateful for every minute of every day as some people claim (usually after a horrible tragedy has befallen them, but from which they have either healed or escaped). Instead, it means that you are strong enough to weather what life sends your way, letting some of the bad stuff roll off your back and grabbing the opportunity to enjoy the good stuff. These things describe people who are emotionally healthy: they are content; they laugh often and have fun; they are able to find and nurture fulfilling relationships; they can effectively balance work and other activities with rest and relaxation; they are able to deal with stress; they can adapt to both planned and unexpected changes; and emotionally healthy people have self-confidence and high self-esteem.

Social health. This is important, and we can describe a person who is socially healthy and another person who needs help in this area, but it is difficult to pull together a definition that covers these ideas. A little research turned up this definition of social health of a person: "that dimension of an individual's well-being that concerns how he gets along with other people, how other people react to him, and how he interacts with social institutions and societal mores." Research has shown that people who are socially involved with their communities recover faster from illnesses and are less affected by symptoms or disabilities.

However, when dealing with the demands of this disease, it is often difficult to turn outward and interact with others. This is especially true when there are big changes to adapt to. Any new or worsening complication may turn my attention inward for a couple of days while I assimilate this new information into my existing concept of who I am. I have also found this happens when there is a big improvement. In the early 1980s, I was one of the "early adopters" of insulin pump technology. Physically, it was great—after years of unpredictable blood sugar swings and feeling pretty miserable, suddenly I felt a little more stable and—dare I say it?—healthy. As great as this was, it was also a huge adjustment—I was so used to being the sick person that I didn't know what to do with my new healthy self. This affected how I perceived myself until I could get my head around the new identity. The outside world, on the other hand, adjusted quickly to my new healthy self and forgot diabetes was still there, which was a little disconcerting, too. Of course, they were quickly and firmly reminded the first time I experienced serious hypoglycemia in their presence.

Many aspects of social health are covered in more detail in Chapter 7. Reform your relationships on your terms.

Make It Better

Don't forget to celebrate your successes. If you improve a symptom or get a good night's sleep for a change, feel proud and reward yourself.

Intellectual health. Intellectual health is characterized by the ability to fluidly think thoughts that incorporate creativity, common sense, and knowledge gained from books and through living. It is the ease in which these aspects of cognition come together in a coherent and appropriate way.

To understand what it is like to experience a lack of intellectual health, think back to when you may have watched 5 straight hours of *Law and Order* or *Seinfeld* reruns. By the end of the television marathon, you feel slower, kind of dazed, drained of energy and lacking the motivation to do much of anything besides eat Cheetos. On the other hand, when you have an intellectually "snappy" kind of day, you get stimulating little mini-rushes of happiness from little endorphin releases in your brain—this might come after giving a good presentation at work, listening to a reading at a bookstore, holding your own in a fast-paced and interesting conversation, or finishing a challenging crossword puzzle.

So, do things to improve your intellectual health. Read a book—better yet, join a book club; listen to a podcast while you are driving; take a class to learn a foreign language; master a new computer program; do a crossword puzzle; pick an issue that you are interested in and research it on the Internet; attend a lecture at the local library or university; watch a foreign-language movie with subtitles, then discuss it with someone—keep your brain active.

Healthy surroundings. Look around you right now. Assuming that you are at home, and not reading this book on a subway, in a mall or on an airplane, you should be able to find a calm place to rest your eyes. Your ears should be soothed by the sounds of silence, nature, or (maybe) tranquil music—if you do hear other people, such as your children, it should be happy sounds of soft laughter and conversation floating to your ears. You shouldn't notice any smells, aside from the occasional light scent of freshly cut grass drifting in your open window.

Okay, seriously. How far does this deviate from your reality? How sad does that make you? Your home should be a lovely retreat where you can relax and recharge. However, most of us probably spend a great deal of mental energy "shutting out" the stress-inducing aspects of our home. Think about what you can do to make at least a small corner of your home more closely resemble a spa-like escape from the outside world—both today (turn off the TV and light a candle) and in the future (paint a room in earth tones and soften the lighting).

Make It Better

Make your home nice. Upgrade your reading chair and rearrange the furniture. The change will do you good.

Spiritual health. Most of the definitions of "spiritual health" or "spirituality" fairly quickly veer down different paths of specific religions or beliefs. While that is where most of us will end up when we think about what these words mean to us, putting out any definition from a specific set of beliefs can only result in excluding some valid ideas about spirituality. Defining spiritual health as the well-being of the soul, that part of a person that is intangible, opens it up to lots of interesting things. I am going to leave the exact meaning of "soul" up to each of you, as, for some people, the soul is an immortal spirit that temporarily inhabits our physical bodies before moving onto another body or place when we die. For others, it is the essence of a person that is basically the sum of who they are, comprised of thoughts, feelings, actions—their personality. Then there are a whole bunch of other definitions in the middle of this spectrum or on other spectrums altogether. Regardless of your take on the matter, it is pretty hard to argue that spiritual health is not important.

To give your spiritual health a boost, try: making a "gratitude" list of all the things (people, places, experiences, books, art, food, basically anything that makes you happy) in your life that you are grateful for and adding one item to it every day, or even just going to a place that inspires you, such as the forest, an art museum, a field of flowers, a cemetery where a relative is buried. Personally I just go to a quiet place to "reconnect" with myself.

Taking these examples of the various aspects of health, here are some for creating health in new places:

Be creative. Think of anything you can do that makes your life better or makes you feel good. Have crazy ideas. Don't limit yourself because of time, money, or other obstacles. Any idea you might have can be broken down into steps. If some of your ideas can't really happen right away, like a vacation or getting a dog, you can get books to research different resorts that you might like to visit, or plan to go to a local dog show to start investigating the different breeds of dogs that might be right for you. Actively thinking about nice things can contribute to health in immeasurable ways.

However, do try some things that are within reach. When choosing activities, make sure you do include some small things that you can accomplish in a day or two. Maybe you'll begin by cleaning up some clutter in your house, or even just clearing the magazines off of the coffee table. Maybe you'll finally get the oil changed in your car so you don't have to think about that anymore. Go to the farmers' market and try a new kind of leafy green vegetable. Health can be found anywhere.

Keep searching for ideas to expand health. Go on a health scavenger hunt throughout the day. Can you make changes to your environment, how you do things, or with whom you do them that will add health to your life?

Do Your Best

Really push yourself to find more health in new places. Do everything you can.

Offset negative thoughts with positive ideas. Try to invest the same amount of time, emotion, and energy into improving your health as you spend thinking about your diabetes. Every time you worry about a new or worsening complication or your long-term prospects, balance that by taking an action to improve your health somewhere. Use your emotional concerns as cues for you to focus on your overall health.

Your Physical Health Is More Than Your Diabetes

Like I mentioned, many of us with diabetes think of our physical health in terms of discomforts or complications that we have. We start with the notion of a flawed body and concentrate on those flaws, rather than thinking about what we can do to feel better.

For many people it is hard to strive for physical wellness when we know that we will never be perfect. For these people, thinking about physical wellness while living with diabetes can be similar to the experience of buying a "perfect" first house, buoyed by fantasies about family meals and romantic moments and wonderful holiday celebrations. However, the home inspection report then gets handed over and bursts that little fantasy bubble, enumerating all of the problems with the soon-to-be new house. It contains items as trivial as leaky faucets and as big as foundation flaws, the accompanying pictures showing details of mold, mildew, rot, possible termite damage, faulty building practices, and places where corners were cut. From that moment on, even years later, one can still look at the personal touches and the love that has gone into this house and occasionally still see that it is icing on top of flaws. Even when everything is clean and organized and the details are just right, gone is the giddy vision of the perfect house.

For some of us, it's hard to learn not to think of our bodies that way. We put the effort in to work out, to eat better, to really take care of ourselves, then remember that there is still more to be done—that the demands of diabetes are relentless. These realizations can take away from the progress that is made and remind us that we will never be perfect, no matter how much we work. The solution is to realize that we should not aim for perfection in pursuing health and wellness, as that is a certain prescription for failure. Instead, the goal of "doing better" in our habits and how we take care of ourselves is a noble—and doable—one.

As people with diabetes, we have extra responsibility when it comes to taking care of our bodies. Most of us living with diabetes are especially aware that it is crucial to keep ourselves as healthy as possible to keep on functioning well.

Strive for Better

I am going to share with you my philosophy for keeping the body going without getting despondent, obsessed, or caught up in circular debates about what is the "right" approach to healthy living: *strive for a little better every day*. That's it, that's all there is to it, but it took me a long time to get here.

> ### Do Your Best
>
> Do everything possible to make today a tiny bit "healthier" than yesterday. Regardless of your diabetes situation, there is a lot of health out there for you to grab.

What do I mean by "strive for a little better every day?" It's very simple. We know on a fundamental level what healthy choices look like: easy things, like salad instead of a Twinkie, a little yoga instead of that third hour of a video game, sleeping instead of doodling around on the Internet at 3:00 AM, and things like that. Yet, in many, maybe most, cases we reject those choices because we like to have a concrete strategy, with specific steps and instructions, rather than relying on our own instincts. We wait to start improving our habits until we find the perfect plan, then we make it an "all or nothing" endeavor. However, it is precisely because the program for "right way to live" often involves complicated exercise programs and diet plans that require huge time commitments and making dramatic changes all at once, that we fail to meet most of the objectives that we had at the beginning of these endeavors. Then we let things slip even more.

Let's start fresh. Let's see what we can do to make the most of what we've got, but still have a good time and maintain our sense of self, and humor, while doing so. Let's tune in a little better to what our bodies and minds instinctively know and take it from there.

With these instructions in mind, there are some fundamental things that we need to do for our physical selves to stay healthy. While "striving for a little better each day," we need to eat (fuel our bodies), get some form of exercise (move our bodies), get enough sleep (rest our bodies), and destress and relax (restore our bodies).

A Note on Eating and Moving

You'll notice that I specifically did not title this section "A Note on Diet and Exercise." You will be disappointed if you have flipped to this section hoping to see a recommendation for a specific diet that will help you control your glucose levels or a prescription for a specific number of minutes of a certain kind of exercise that you "should" do a certain number of times each week. That ain't my department and there is no specific diet or prescription for exercise.

The main idea here is to find a way to stay motivated in the face of the relentless demands and chronic nature of diabetes. We are pretty much all aware that the experts say "diets" fail in over 95% of people who lose weight because once the weight is lost, the person goes back to their old ways. There is no finish line, like a goal number on the scale, to cross in diabetes. Therefore, it is crucial that we incorporate our diabetes-friendly lifestyle into our lives with diabetes.

I'll share what works for me. It may seem like I have strong willpower and determination, as I stick to my workout routine pretty well. However, in my opinion, people have it all wrong. People think discipline is about making choices, the "right" choice or the "hard" choice. It is actually the exact opposite—discipline is about removing choices. For example, on certain days my alarm goes off at 5:10 AM, and I get on my stationary bicycle. If I were to ask myself, "Do I want to get up and get on the bike today?" thus introducing an option when that alarm goes off, there is about a 50% chance (or less) that I will actually go through with it. If, instead, I mentally remove the idea there is a choice, then I will just get up and do it.

I do the same thing with food. I only eat salads or soup for lunch most days during the week, period. If I walk into a meeting and there is pizza, it is as if it doesn't exist for me. If I had not set my salad/soup rule in stone with myself, then I would likely look at the pizza and have to make a choice about what I was going to do. After a great deal of internal negotiation, I would likely end up having a piece. Don't get me wrong—I do eat pizza at other times. However, designating specific days as those when choices are removed makes it much easier for me to stick to what is healthy.

That is what works for me. Feel free to borrow it or create your own internal laws. It just seems like there is certainly enough stuff for us to deal with that we don't need to be having long, tiring conversations with ourselves that often end with disappointment. Life is too short, really.

Fuel Your Body

Mostly I just want to talk to you about making wise choices about what you put into your body, then turn the project over to you. This is an area where recommendations for people with type 1 diabetes and those with type 2 diabetes vary, so I would highly recommend talking to a certified diabetes educator or nutritionist to get a handle on how you are going to approach food as a person with diabetes. You may be someone who wants pretty firm guidelines, and a professional can help you find the best strategy for you. There are many ways to organize your thoughts to get the right amounts of the right foods in a way that is understandable and is not too restrictive. Some of the approaches include counting carbohydrates, counting calories, using exchange lists, using the "plate method," or using the diabetes food pyramid. There will also be general principles to be applied, and you will need to know about things like the glycemic index, approximate grams of carbohydrates in different foods, and portion sizes.

Let me reiterate—it is important to visit a professional who has experience and knowledge in this area. Ideally that would be a registered dietician who is a certified diabetes educator, an RD/CDE. The vast majority of us, diabetes or not, have a great deal of confusion around food. How could they not when there is so much contradictory advice being thrown around? We are told to eat more fish, for example, only to encounter reams of information about toxic mercury content, unsafe fish farming practices, certain species of fish forced onto the endangered species list and inappropriate antibiotic use in fish. We are told at the same time that eggs are both bad for you and good for you. And, I am pretty positive that more than a few social occasions have been ruined by overly zealous people getting into the "low-carb" vs. "low-fat" debate.

However, even before we get help from a RD/CDE, most of us have the basic knowledge and instincts to be able to eat in a way that does not harm us. When we approach food, there are a couple of things that we can do so that we don't feel worse, and that would be a huge improvement indeed for many people.

Cultivate good eating habits. While what we eat is clearly important, *how* we eat is often the culprit to eating too much and making poor food choices. Many of us stuff food in while sitting in front of the TV, messing around on the computer, driving our cars, or doing any number of things that distract us from exactly what and how much is going in our mouths. Here are a couple of things to experiment with to bring this under control, and make eating a more mindful (and dignified) activity: only eat while sitting at a table; when you eat, eat—don't multitask; try putting your fork down between bites and focus on the food that you are chewing.

Do Your Best

Eat to feel physically good 15 minutes after you stop eating. Eat for your body. However, eat to enjoy, as well.

Just saying. . . Okay, I don't want to spew a bunch of rules, but there are a couple of truisms that it never hurts to be reminded of. Michael Pollan, author of *In Defense of Food: An Eater's Manifesto* and *An Omnivore's Dilemma*, implores us to "Eat food. Not too much. Mostly plants." This pretty much sums it up, especially if you are a little thoughtful in your definition of "food," to the exclusion of things that are made entirely in laboratories or that in no way resemble anything that people ate a century ago.

Do Your Best

"Eat food. Not too much. Mostly plants."
                                                                    —*Michael Pollan*

Move Your Body

Study after study after study shows that exercise is critical to people with diabetes for so many reasons, including lowering blood pressure and LDL cholesterol, helping insulin to work better, and improving circulation, among other benefits. But exercising can also introduce challenges to managing glucose levels, especially if you have type 1 diabetes.

If you have never exercised regularly, or it has been a long time, this is something that you may want to discuss with a CDE, who can help you come up with an appropriate plan. The ideal approach to exercise would be a plan that would keep you interested and be challenging enough to have results, but not so intensive that you get too tired, too sore or too discouraged to continue. That can come through trial and error, and a professional should be able to assess your interests and abilities to find just the right balance. Oh, yeah—it goes without saying that you need your doctor's clearance before starting any exercise program.

Do Your Best

Get more energy by exercising. No, really—try it and see for yourself.

The daily 15. By doing something physical every day, you can quickly build a daily habit of moving more. You can start by simply scheduling 15 minutes each day for activity. Over the course of a couple of weeks, you can gradually increase that time by 2 minutes every day pretty painlessly to get to 30 minutes, and experiment with different types and intensities of physical activity. Your activity doesn't have to be traditional exercise—you can garden, do housework with vigor, stretch—whatever gets your body moving.

Rest Your Body

You need to sleep. More specifically, you need to sleep between 7 and 9 hours each night. Not only is adequate sleep an important component of how good we feel during the day, it has also been shown that too little sleep can make it harder to control blood sugar.[1] Experts think this is due to higher levels of cortisol circulating in the bloodstream, which makes the body more resistant to insulin. In addition, sleep deprivation leads to decreased amounts of leptin (appetite suppressant) and increased amounts of ghrelin (appetite stimulant), a combination which may drive people to eat more and less healthy than they would like.[2]

The first thing to try, of course, is working with your doctor to address any symptom that is keeping you awake. Some things can be treated effectively and easily with medications and it is worth a try.

The next strategy involves various approaches to improving your "sleep hygiene." Sleep hygiene is often overlooked, as most people think that sleep is something that your body should just be able to do, like breathing. In order to fall asleep fast and stay asleep, you may need to retrain your body. Here are some things to try:

Use your bed only for sleeping. If you read, watch TV, or even think in bed, you are telling your body that something other than sleep needs to be done. This is confusing to the primitive parts of our brain that control basic bodily functions like sleep. In order to retrain your body, you are going to have to send only one message each night: "It's time to sleep." What you are going to do is simple: wait until you are tired, then lie down and try to sleep. If you can't fall asleep within 15 minutes, get up and do something really boring and calming, using dim lights only. Try to go to sleep again when you feel tired. For those of you who have been fretting since reading the heading of this paragraph, don't worry—sex is an approved bed activity that can help you sleep better.

Make It Better

Do everything possible to fix your sleep. Poor sleep makes everything worse.

Light and dark. This one is also pretty easy. Make sure that you are exposed to sunlight during the day and that you dim the lights as night approaches. The reasons for this are simple—what makes you fall asleep are changes in the level of the hormone melatonin circulating in your body. During the day, light stimulates a part of the brain, known as the *suprachiasmatic nucleus*, which tells the pineal gland to decrease the melatonin level when it is light out and to increase it when it is dark. The brighter the light, the bigger the decrease of melatonin, and the darker the dark, the bigger the increase.

Avoid sleep thieves. There are four of them: caffeine, alcohol, stress, and nicotine. Caffeine, which is a stimulant, keeps the body alert and energized. Your body can process 50% of a cup of coffee in 6 hours (the half-life of caffeine). This week, have no caffeine in the 6 hours before you go to sleep, including chocolate and tea. Using alcohol to fall asleep will keep you from having deep dream cycles of sleep, as well as cause blood sugar spikes at inconvenient times, both of which will wake you up. A glass of wine with dinner is fine if you are going to be up for a few more hours, as your body takes about an hour per drink to process the alcohol. That means if you want to drink two glasses of wine, you should be finished at least 2 hours before going to bed. Stress will interfere with your ability to fall asleep by sending a message to your brain that there is something important to be doing other than sleeping. As for nicotine. . . Among other reasons to quit smoking, a study at Johns Hopkins showed that smokers are four times more likely to complain of poor sleep quality than nonsmokers.

Have a nightly ritual. Your body loves habits. By creating a habit that is strongly associated with sleep, your body will know exactly what to do when you lie down in bed. Decide what you would like to do during your ritual. Some people like to read in a comfortable chair for a few minutes. Other like to just stretch, brush their teeth and be calm. A warm bath or shower can help get you into that relaxation zone. Changing the scent in your bedroom can also be very helpful, because your sense of smell is tightly linked to the emotional control centers of the brain. Like Pavlov's dog, you can train yourself to feel sleepy by simply smelling a certain smell when you are tired. Try lighting a scented candle or using a lavender-scented pillow or room spray. The important thing is to repeat the same ritual every night to establish cues that tell your body it is time to sleep.

Restore Your Body

Being stressed is unhealthy for anyone. It drains your energy, worsens your sleep, and damages your long-term health. It also looks like stress can lead to or worsen relapses.

There are several things you can do to reduce stress, but one of the easiest ones with instant benefits is meditation. In fact, most of the other stress-reducing techniques have a meditative component at their core: prayer, music therapy, art therapy, creative visualization, and even mindfully performing everyday tasks, like folding laundry or preparing dinner.

Meditation can reduce stress, decrease negative emotions, increase creativity, and promote good health, all while helping you live more mindfully and deliberately. You can also benefit from meditation if you are interested in establishing more control over your emotions, as well as cultivating your mental skills and increasing your ability to concentrate.

Make It Better

Meditation is great—it trains the brain to quiet down and focus. We could *all* (with or without diabetes) use help with that.

Meditation is not about making your brain stop thinking—that is impossible. It's more about letting the "noise" die down by not engaging with the thoughts that come and letting them drift past. Give it a try.

Here's how to meditate:

Schedule a time. Schedule 5 minutes each day this week to sit and focus. This should be the same time every day. Make sure that you will not be interrupted by anything during this time—no phones and no knocks on the door.

Sit. Sit comfortably in an alert position. You can sit in a chair or on a cushion placed on the floor—it does not matter. Make your back as straight as possible. Keep your head level and look slightly downward. Pick one spot on the wall and stare at it. Your intention is only to sit—so no looking around the room. If you want, you can close your eyes, but try not to fall asleep. Put your hands anywhere that is comfortable.

Focus. Choose one of the following to focus on:

- Pick a word that has some meaning to you like "peace," "quiet" or "calm." Repeat that word slowly to yourself as you sit.

- Count your breaths. Every time you exhale, count. When you get to "ten," return to "one."

That's pretty much it. Try it a couple of times and experience the benefits for yourself.

The Bottom Line

Take a minute and think of some of the people that you know. Let's start with that guy (we all know one of these) who has no physical disabilities, a stable financial situation, a family that seems to like each other well enough and are all healthy, and a nice house. Still, nothing is ever good enough; he is convinced that everything (including the weather and the economy) and everyone (including the President of the United States) are aligned specifically against *him*. He is, slowly but surely, accumulating all sorts of health problems from stress.

Then consider someone else you might know who lives with a much more challenging situation. Many of us know someone who is living with challenges so big that we shake our heads and say, "I don't know how he (or she) does it." However, many of these people are delightful to be around and seem to have a lion's share of happiness and contentment. Sure, they can get down at times, occasionally even overwhelmed. However, these feelings do not taint the rest of their outlook on life. They see the good in everyone, the beauty that exists in the world. They grab chances to enjoy life. Even if their circumstances are objectively much worse than ours at any given moment, our encounters with these people bring us lightness and laughs. We are energized by these people, and the world is a happier place with them in it. These people cultivate "health" every day, in everything they do— even as their situation remains difficult.

So, which type of person do you want to know, and more importantly, who do you want to be?

7

Reform Relationships on Your Terms

Because I have been living with diabetes since I was 12 years old, I do not really have a "before diabetes" and "after diabetes" perspective on relationships.

Of course, I can talk about various social challenges that diabetes introduced at different points in my life—however, they are not all unique—all of us have the unrelenting desire to fit in as teenagers and few of us really do fit in for one reason or another. All of us bring our own special baggage and impediments to our adult relationships. Those of us with chronic illnesses do not have a corner on the market of relationship challenges.

That being said, there are some interpersonal moments that are specific to diabetes. While many people these days are reliant on portable technology like smartphones that they check compulsively, most people are not being directly monitored by their gadgets, with beeps and lights alerting the outside world to their bodies' workings or malfunctions. Also, no one can bring a festive party to a screeching halt like a person with diabetes reaching for a donut.

Perhaps the most global impact of diabetes on any relationship, casual or close, is the judgment that we feel coming our way. For people like me with type 1 diabetes, I feel this with each complication—the faulty equation that tight blood glucose control automatically equals a life free of complications, working to bring people to the conclusion that I did these things to myself through neglect or recklessness in pursuit of a good time. Despite the fact that it is illogical to think that I woke up one day with the thought "Hey, sitting still so that my retina can be burned by lasers sounds like great fun," the sympathy that comes my way from many people when complications emerge is limited and conditional.

People with type 2 diabetes have it even worse, as the outside world has decided that they "brought the whole diabetes thing" upon themselves through gluttony, laziness, or other undesirable traits.

For these reasons, people with diabetes often end up hiding big things in relationships. We may hide our behaviors for fear that our actions may be perceived as harmful or not good enough. We may hide our fears about complications in order to avoid advice and hollow-sounding (and possibly rage-inducing) encouragement to "Try harder! You can beat this!" We may hide our confusing and disappointing test results because we don't really want to engage with others in a hunt for clues as to what we "did wrong" and strategies to help us "do better." While usually well-meaning, this type of feedback is incredibly isolating.

I force myself to wear my diabetes on the outside, along with my monitors and pump, so that I can quickly react to keep this type of judgment at bay. I do not love this role. I often feel self-conscious. I do not enjoy conversations that I am not in control of. In my job as Senior Product Manager in Diabetes Marketing at a large pharmaceutical company, I try to represent other people with diabetes and how they might react to or perceive something, but really do not relish sharing details about my own diabetes with people at work.

There is no doubt that one of the worst aspects of diabetes can be, for many people, how it impacts them socially. All human relationships are complicated, but the intrusion of diabetes, with its often invisible symptoms and incessant demands, can strain marriages, friendships, family interactions, and workplace dealings. While many of these problems come from the other people, it is often us, the people with diabetes, that are contributing most to the awkwardness and strife, by not feeling comfortable with how to present our diabetes to the outside world.

Give Diabetes an Appropriate Role in Your Relationships

Here's a newsflash, in case you hadn't noticed: Diabetes can change dynamics in a relationship. These changes can exacerbate problems in relationships, or they can make relationships stronger. They can be subtle differences, like a concerned glance from your spouse, lingering an extra second when you seem to be losing track of your thoughts, wondering if you may be hypoglycemic. They can be dramatic changes: being avoided by a friend who is uncomfortable because you have checked blood glucose or injected insulin during a lunch date, or conversely, suddenly having an acquaintance blossom into a very good friend after she came to your rescue during a scary complication, as my friend Veronica became an emotional lifeline when I was battling cardiac neuropathy. An intimate relationship may take on a new dimension when a dramatic blood glucose drop brings a sexual encounter to an ill-timed halt.

Here is another secret that I will let you in on: People are complex, so complex that they often do not understand their own actions. This often results in their being unpredictable. In relationships, diabetes can make things feel "weird." In many circumstances this can be avoided and we can keep our relationships healthy. However, and this is a huge "however," you cannot control other people's thoughts or actions, no matter what you do. It is up to us to do what we can to control ourselves and conduct ourselves in a dignified or loving manner in our dealings with others. That is what each of us can do—be the person that we would want to befriend.

Take Charge

Decide how you want to talk about diabetes in each of your relationships. Take control of the dialog and deliberately create the relationship you want between your people and your diabetes.

All of us have different roles in the various relationships we are in, including those of daughter/son, spouse, parent, co-worker or friend. Just as each of these roles comes with unique modes of interaction and places in a hierarchy, our diabetes can impact each type of relationship differently. The uncertainty and changing stresses that come with this disease can lead to fear, resentment, stress, or loneliness in both the person with diabetes and the other parties. However, handled strategically, the various relationships in your life can be protected from the negative impacts of diabetes to a great degree.

You (Person With Diabetes) as a Spouse/Partner

As trite as it may sound, diabetes can strengthen relationships as couples strategize how to work together as a team to compensate for the effects of diabetes. However, marriage and long-term relationships can be difficult for healthy people in the best of circumstances, and diabetes can certainly introduce impediments that change the whole vision of what both partners "signed up for." The person without diabetes may become the primary breadwinner or have to take on more parenting tasks during hard times.

The spouse or partner of a person with diabetes may also find that they are gradually (or suddenly) taking on a caregiving role. This may start out with little things, such as helping figure out food counts. However, it can progress into providing more intimate kinds of help, like administering injections or assisting with hygiene needs at crucial times. In this way, diabetes can transform a partnership between lovers to more of a parent-child situation, stripping people of dignity and introducing embarrassment and dependence, even though that is not intended.

The "collateral damage" from this shift in roles can be the death of a once-healthy sex life. Further alienation can occur when the person with diabetes begins to perceive themselves to be a burden, feels guilty, or stops talking to their partner about how they feel: in short, shutting them out emotionally, while making more demands on them physically.

At the risk of sounding trite (again), many of these problems can be avoided through good communication. Your partner needs to know how you are feeling, needs to know that their efforts are noticed—that all the work they are putting in is not going into a black hole. Your partner also needs to know that you are there for them, even if they need to vent about your diabetes or discuss their own diabetes-related fears and emotions—in this case it is your job to listen. You both can take advantage of days, or even minutes, when the diabetes is less "intrusive" or more predictable to enjoy your relationship through talking, laughing, and having sex.

The Real World

You can't blame diabetes for who you are or for who your partner is. Diabetes puts extra tension on relationships but doesn't change the fundamentals. You are still you and your partner is still your partner.

I am not unrealistic. If you are involved with a selfish pig, diabetes will surely not change that, and may speed up the demise of the relationship. Also, sometimes even good people cannot handle what their partner's diabetes has thrown at them, and a relationship that might be okay in wonderful circumstances will falter under this kind of stress.

The most important ingredients in a relationship are honesty, caring, and dignity. These will take you far, even far enough to be out of the long reach of diabetes.

You (Person With Diabetes) as a Parent

I can tell you with certainty that young children pick up on the fact that something is wrong when a parent is not feeling well. This can manifest as increased clinginess, regression in terms of speech or potty-training progress, or reversion to younger behavior (such as needing a pacifier). Children who are a little older may get worried that something terrible is happening—that their parent will die, that they will die, that they did something terrible and whatever is going on is their fault. This may turn into sleeping issues or nightmares, withdrawing emotionally, or acting out at school.

Teenagers may be embarrassed about the whole situation, making them (even more) resentful and difficult to get along with. They may also go in the other direction, taking on emotional and physical responsibilities that put them in a caretaking or parent-type role.

The Real World

Don't forget that your children are entitled to their own reactions and emotions about your diabetes. While it is your diabetes, it is also your family's diabetes.

Everyone with children has to make their own way as parents. I can't tell you what to do; I cannot tell you that you must be open about your diabetes with your children or that you should hide the scary parts from them. I know that many people are uncomfortable with either approach, and I understand. The "experts" (most of whom do *not* have diabetes) say that we should answer all questions about our diabetes honestly and directly, adjusting the information as the kids get older. That might, or might not, work for you. I know that some people choose to keep their diabetes from their children until they reach a certain age or something happens where it must be revealed, the thinking being that they are letting their children have a good shot at a normal life, without the pervasive worry of having a sick parent.

Mostly I think kids react to things the way they see us react to things. In my opinion, if you teach kids about hypoglycemia, not only are they less likely to freak out if they see you experience this, they may actually be able to help. However, this involves talking with them about the whole subject before you are in this situation.

The only thing I can tell you with 100% clarity is that it is impossible to show your children too much love.

We also need to remember that as parents to grown children who no longer live with us, we are still their parents, even if this relationship has come to closely resemble (or becomes) a friendship. We may require more help than before, but it is important to avoid leaning on our children too much emotionally and telling them intimate details of our life better saved for our spouse, a close friend, or a therapist.

Person With Diabetes as a Child

Since I was diagnosed at age 12, I have an interesting perspective on the impact of a diabetes diagnosis on a parent; I was old enough at diagnosis to remember things, yet still under the complete care of my parents. An interesting twist on our family's situation was that I was not the first—my brother Ed had been diagnosed at the same age just 2 years before, at which time the doctors assured Mom and Dad that there was no possible way to have more than one kid with type 1 diabetes in the family. Backed by these promises, all of my symptoms were chalked up to a vitamin C deficiency and I was sent to bed with a big glass of orange juice and told to get some rest.

When it became clear that I did, in fact, have type 1 diabetes, my parents just became more determined that we would all deal with this unwelcome news in a proactive way. Mom insisted that I learn how to self-inject before I left the hospital that first time. My parents spent scarce family finances on diet sodas, fresh fruits and vegetables, doctor appointments, insulin, and myriad other things that it takes to live with diabetes. My parents' mantra around our diabetes was that this disease would not hold us back. We would be independent and we would keep going. So we did.

However, I know that this disease took a toll on my parents. Like any parents, they wanted us to fit in, to be happy, to have normal lives.

For all the talk of independence, Mom would give me my shot before school and on those days where I simply could not bring myself to do it. They hid their fear and stress from us, but it must have been terrifying—the tools were rudimentary and the prognosis different than what it is now.

For those of you in the position of being a grown-up that faces the task of telling your parents that you have diabetes, I'll tell you something that may surprise you—this time, for a little while, your diabetes is not about you. If you are a parent, you know that you would much sooner take on any pain before allowing your child to experience just a fraction of the discomfort. It is no different for your parents, even though you are all grown up.

So, be gentle. Be understanding. Have your facts ready. Be calm. Try not to get upset when the tears come. Try to be patient when you hear the latest suggestion for a freaky remedy or hear something about diabetes that was on the evening news or in *Reader's Digest* repeated back to you for the tenth time. Your parent is trying to understand and help in their way. Don't shut them out, but do what you can to bring them to terms with your situation.

You also need to realize that if your parent also has diabetes, there may be an element of guilt from the genetic nature of the disease, with your mom or dad convinced that it is their fault that you have diabetes. Without deconstructing this too much, decide how you are going to deal with this—listen to as much as you can, then tell them it is time to deal with what it is. Do put limits around this subject if you start getting annoyed—after all, you have a new reality to grapple with.

The Real World

Let people "borrow" your diabetes for a while and talk about how it impacts them.

Person With Diabetes as a Sibling, Close Friend or an Acquaintance

Again, I have a pretty rare perspective on telling a sibling that you have diabetes, as my brother paved the way for me with his diagnosis 2 years earlier. In many ways, Ed was my lifeline in those early months and years. I recall a day, just 1 year after my diagnosis, when a strange sensation on my legs—as if water was running down them—had me worried and scared. I mentioned this to Ed, who said he often felt the same thing. We later understood that this was peripheral neuropathy, but at that time all we knew was that it was weird, it was scary, and we didn't like it. We also knew, however, that we were not alone—we had each other.

You know who the people in your life are that you absolutely *need* to tell and for which reasons (she is your sister; he is your ex-husband who might need to take care of your child for a while if you have an acute medical situation; she is your confidant to whom you tell everything).

Then there are a whole bunch of people who you might want to tell about your diabetes, or not, or just a little bit about it. Take each person on a case-by-case basis. Some people you might want to tell because they went through health problems themselves and your gut tells you that they would be a wonderful source of support. Knowing about your diabetes might jointly benefit you and the other person in different ways—your child's teacher might be able to help him work through some worried or scared feelings he has about Mommy being in the hospital, or the neighbor could accept deliveries of diabetes supplies while you are at work. Then there are people who simply don't need to know, unless there is an extreme situation. You know who they are. Do not feel compelled to share all of your information with everyone, especially if it can be somehow used in a negative manner.

Person With Diabetes as a Potential Romantic Interest

Dating is like going through puberty or being a brand-new mother—it can be terrifying (and terrible at times), but if you make it through okay, the rewards might be really good. If you are a person with diabetes who is at the early (or embryonic) stages of a relationship, you have two choices: 1) tell the other person about your diabetes, or 2) don't tell the other person about your diabetes. Of course, the loveliest outcome would be that you would tell the person, and they would say, "Oh, okay. That is no big deal, considering how fabulous, funny, and beautiful you are. What can I do to help?" Once we wake up from that fantasy, we worry about the following outcomes: (1) you tell the other person and it scares them away, or (2) you don't tell the other person and you are keeping a secret, which will either come out later or the relationship will perish before the truth is revealed.

I wish I could tell you what to do. You are pretty much on your own with this one, as we all have different personalities and find different types of partners interesting or desirable. What might have worked for me may not be a good idea for you. I will offer my opinion on one thing, however. We all pretty much know how a first date is going within about 15 minutes. Give it 30 minutes and we can guess with about 93% accuracy if we will see this person again. If you are thinking "probably not," there is really no need to say anything about the diabetes. If you are feeling the "vibe," I see no problem in mentioning it, despite the advice that you might get from "dating experts" (whoever those people are). I really think that if a person is going to be "scared away," it will happen whether you tell them right away or after several dates. I also think if you wait longer than the aforementioned several dates to tell them, they may get nervous about a relationship because you were not honest from the beginning. On the other hand, your diabetes can be an excellent "loser screener," as another date following your diabetes disclosure indicates that this person may have excellent potential to become more serious.

Disclose Your Diabetes With Class (and Compassion)

Disclosure is a little difficult for me to address constructively. Because I have lived with diabetes since childhood, all of the people who are close to me know about it. Circumstances in my work frequently put me in a situation of disclosure as if it is part of the job description. The people whom I encounter in different situations and settings need not worry about being left out of the loop—they will soon be clued in when something attached to me beeps, buzzes, or flashes in their presence, requiring my attention (and usually an explanation).

However, the majority of people with diabetes are diagnosed as adults and have a variety of preexisting relationships. Although many may be reluctant to tell others about their diabetes (usually because of the real or perceived judgment mentioned at the beginning of this chapter), there may be some very practical reasons to bring people up to speed.

For instance, you will almost certainly find yourself making conscious and complicated choices about food, especially in the beginning, when the carb counting and glycemic index algorithms are still fuzzy. You do not need people urging you to eat things or jokingly refilling your plate or wine glass. On a more acute level, you may actually need help in a hypoglycemic "situation"—needless to say, this is *not* an ideal time to disclose your diabetes status.

Take Charge

Know what your goal is when you talk about your diabetes. Are you looking for sympathy? For support? Do you just want to shock someone? Make sure your communication and goals are linked to each other.

Here are some tips to make disclosing your diabetes status more palatable to you and the person you are telling:

Avoid shocking people (unless you want to). Set up this part of the conversation a little. Start by saying something like, "there is something that I would like to share with you because you are my friend." While this may seem a little staged, it is better than, "Sit down. This is serious. Are you sitting down?"

Use details. Part of reducing the shock factor is the use of relevant details. If you simply tell someone that you have diabetes, they are left to fill in these details themselves, and (trust me) the first things that come to mind are sad and scary images from news stories of people who died from diabetes or a friend's uncle who was a double amputee at an early age. If you tell your story—including your freaky symptoms, your suspicions that something was wrong, and the funny or creepy doctors that you encountered—you give the other person something to relate to. They can get involved with the narrative and picture you going through these things. The diabetes then becomes part of the story, not a shocking bomb that is dropped.

Tell with feeling. Be sure to use a lot of energy—positive and/or negative—in your story. This will allow your listener to see how the diabetes is affecting you and how to gauge their own reaction.

Make your listeners characters in your story. Maybe they helped you a few times when you were tired. Maybe you yelled at them when feeling stressed. Maybe you want to ask them for help in the event of hypoglycemia or if you need a procedure. Including them in the story will not only hold their interest, but it will also open up the possibility of them being part of your story in the future. This will also open up the story into a dialogue and allow them to ask questions of their own.

Use These Communication "Cheat Sheets"

It's a terrible situation, and one that I have found myself in far too often. You feel awful, and want to communicate that to a loved one, but you feel too awful to find the right words, so you use the wrong words. A fight or misunderstanding occurs, which makes you feel more awful for all new and different reasons.

We have words to explain every nuance, every shade of gray, with incredible precision and artistry. That is, until you are really desperate to get your point across because you are under physical and emotional duress from one diabetes symptom or another—at the time that you need to explain things accurately and concisely, in a way that people will understand and react with empathy, your words seem to abandon you.

I find myself lying awake at night and replaying many conversations, using the words I wish I could have found at the moment that I needed them. I decided to do us all a favor and put down some of these thoughts for us to use at critical moments. Feel free to read from the book, to point to the paragraphs, to write it out in your own words, adapting to make it just right. If you feel strange about using a stranger's words to "talk" to your loved ones, think about the greeting card aisle on Valentine's Day and all those big, shambly men reading dozens of cards until they find just the right one to communicate "I love you" to someone they see every day. Hallmark knows that we all need a little help sometimes—they just haven't gotten around to making the diabetes greeting card line yet, so I went ahead and did it for them (with fewer rhymes and no smiling puppy or laughing kitten illustrations).

"I don't feel good."

Saying the words 'I don't feel good' isn't really accurate. That is because the right words to describe exactly how I feel don't seem to exist. Attempts to put words to it might come across to you as overly dramatic, exaggerated or maudlin—and knowing you thought that I was any of those things would only make me feel worse.

Let's keep it at this: When I feel this way, my limitations define me in many ways. I [am unable to think clearly, I am dizzy, I am nauseated]. I cannot fake my way through feeling like this. I am depleted and these are the times that I have to admit, even to myself, that I am not entirely whole or healthy.

I am telling you this because I want you to know about this aspect of diabetes, which, unfortunately is also a part of me. This will not last forever. I will have times, hopefully soon, when I feel intact again. I will be more functional. Until then, I need acceptance. I know that this is also frustrating and scary to you, and you are not forgotten.

Do Your Best

Practice your communication. There may be big difference between what you think you said, what you actually said, and how someone understood what you said. Words like "tired" or "bad day" may have very different meanings when spoken by someone with diabetes. Be sure to communicate what you mean.

"I am sad/angry."

I know all of it—I know that there are people that have it worse than me. I know that being angry or sad doesn't 'help' me get better, whatever that means. I know that it's not considered healthy to wallow in negative feelings.

I also know that I don't really care about all of that right now (and maybe don't even believe it all). Diabetes has stolen something, many things, from me. I am angry and sad about the things I have lost (feeling good, living carefree, being 'normal') and the things that I have gained (physical pain, worry about getting worse, daily reminders that I am living with a chronic and unpredictable disease).

I am not blaming anyone for these feelings, although that would be easier. I am sorry if I lash out at you or turn away from you. I need to battle with these things right now. I will come back. I need patience more than anything, and a little space to finish this round of the fight.

I also know that you may be sad and angry, too. Let's both try to remember that it's the diabetes, and not us, that is the cause of these feelings.

"I just can't right now."

I want to, I really do. I would love to [fill in the blank] more than you know. I know it would be good for me to leave the house/be with people/have fun. I want to be like a 'normal person' and make plans and keep them. I want little outings to be fun and not fill me with dread, wondering how bad I will feel and spending time strategizing how to make it through the situation or get out of it gracefully. I want to be the person who grabs her sweater or binoculars or sunglasses and says, 'Come on! Let's go! What are you waiting for?' as I beat you out the door.

However, I just can't right now. I'm sorry. Maybe next time. Ask me again, please.

"I love you."

I love you.

I cannot count the number of times that I attempted to write (then erased) this particular little helper script for us all. I finally came to the realization that these simple words will do the trick if they are said in a heartfelt way, and that adding in additional verbiage about diabetes or pain or being sorry that you have diabetes just messes up the whole thing somehow. It helps to be holding the person's hand and looking directly into their eyes when you say it. You can also pick up the phone and achieve pretty much the same effect, as long as there is no TV on, children competing for attention or dinner that needs constant stirring on the stove—just you and the other person connecting for long enough to tell them these words.

By the way, I recommend the same technique for saying "Thank you."

A Special Note—"Help Now!"

For all the advice and scripts and pushes to "just communicate what you need," there will be moments that you urgently require help, only to find that your power of communication has completely left you and that you are feeling woozy from hypoglycemia. I recommend that you discuss this situation with your spouse, close friend, or loved ones and come up with a code word that means "Help now!" Think of something that does not sound too alarming to other people, but rather just lets the other person know that they are needed. For instance, I might forgo using "Code red!" or "Situation critical!" in lieu of a cute little secret code phrase. Remember, the goal is to get the help you need right away without making anyone too flustered. The discussion about why you need help and your emotions around the situation can come later.

Assess People

We all have people in our lives. Some of these people are helpful and some are not. Some understand what it is like to have a chronic illness like diabetes, some do not. Some people make us feel better, and others make us feel worse. We often don't realize the impact people have on us or our diabetes until things blow up or we have spent too much time feeling bad about ourselves, not realizing that maybe we don't need certain people in our lives. Conversely, we may take supportive people for granted, just because they have always been there for us and we neglect to give them the attention that they deserve. At some point it is good to take a close objective-as-possible look at the people in our lives and decide if we need to change the relationship in some way.

Take Charge

Try to make the most helpful people the ones that you deal with regularly. Don't leave any social support that is available to you untapped.

By answering a few targeted questions about the people in your life, you'll create an opportunity to discover how these relationships impact your diabetes. This will help you determine what actions to take in order to construct a social environment for yourself that increases your health. Without taking the time to think about how the people around you impact your diabetes, you may be creating or perpetuating negative situations or missing opportunities for support.

Here are your steps to assessing people:

Make a list. Make a list of the important people in your life. List every-one, even people that you have a connection with but do not see regu-larly. Also, be sure to list people that you see once a week or more (co-workers, people from church, people in a club). Include all the people you talk with on the phone, communicate with by e-mail, or chat with online.

Score them. For each person, decide how supportive that person would be in a crisis, on a scale of 1 to 10. You would give a "1" to a person who makes things worse, and a "10" to a person who is completely and utterly helpful and supportive, with most people falling somewhere in the middle. Place the person's "score" to the left of their name. You can leave a blank next to anyone you feel like you don't know well enough, but try to make a guess about how they would respond if you called on them for help. Also, remember that some of the most helpful people are the ones that help you forget about the disease for a while, not just those who help with diabetes-related needs.

Score them again. Next, give each of the people a score, on a scale of 1 to 10, based on how much you talk to these people about your diabetes or other problems. Write this number to the right of the name. People you talk to the most about your diabetes and problems get a "10," and people to whom you've never mentioned your diabetes or other prob-lems get a "1," with most people receiving scores between these two extremes.

Assess your people. Look over your list. Do the people with a "10" on the left also have a "10" on the right? Are the people who are most support-ive the ones you talk with about your diabetes? If the lists don't look the same, you may have a great deal of untapped support.

Make a plan. For each of the people who scored high on the "support-ive" list (the one to the left of the name), write out one thing they can do to help you right now or in the future. Maybe they could help relieve your stress. Maybe you could spend an afternoon with them just hav-ing fun. Maybe they are good at searching the Internet for information.

Maybe they would just be good at listening to you. For each person, find one thing they could do to help.

You need to be able to rely on people and know they will be there for you. You might ask someone just to respond to a question by e-mail, to tell their story about how they coped with something difficult in their own life, or to help you more directly. Look over your list or come up with something new. For a little challenge, ask at least three different people to do one thing this week. Practice asking for help.

Tips for Increasing Social Support

You don't have to directly ask people for help—some people do it naturally. Just pick up the phone and talk with someone about what is on your mind. That counts.

Many people say they are afraid to be a burden, but often what is behind that is the fear of exposing oneself. Diabetes can be scary, but if you keep all of your emotions about it bottled up inside, you can blow the scariness out of proportion. Instead talk with people who are supportive. They can help keep your thoughts and feelings about your diabetes in perspective.

Get Help

No one can help if you don't ask. Be considerate, specific, and respectful when you ask for help and people will gladly pitch in.

Don't overlook people. You may be surprised how helpful an occasional acquaintance, a co-worker, or a friend from church can be. By talking about your diabetes and asking for help, you are reaching out and making a connection. If you just keep answering "Fine" in response to the question "How are you?" you are shutting people out.

Don't just complain to people. It's not about getting sympathy—it's about getting help with the things you need. Be sure to figure out how to return the help and make the relationship mutual.

Make an effort to increase your social support. Take time this week to reconnect with old friends, to get out more, and to meet new people. Spend time thinking about ways you can increase the number of people you come into contact with. Find organizations to join and people to spend time with. Don't do things alone, call and invite people to come with you. Spend some real effort here—you never know whom you might meet or when a so-so friendship might mature into something wonderful.

Take Care of Your Caregivers

I am pretty reluctant to throw the word "caregiver" around, as it conjures up images of people caring for others who are bedridden or have frank dementia and require full-time care to get basic needs met. However, the people closest to us *are* often taking care of us to varying degrees.

My partner Nancy helps me on a daily basis with humor and a matter-of-fact way of looking at situations. The most memorable moments have been when I am at my lowest emotional and physical points because of a complication. Nancy knows how to break things down into very nonthreatening steps. When I was temporarily blind in one eye and the time had come to go to my retinologist and make a final decision about a vitrectomy, I was in no way ready to deal with any of it. Nancy got me from one point to the next, then to the next, and so on, by saying, "Right now, all you have to do is get in the car." At the doctor's office she said, "Okay, now all you have to think about is getting more information. That's all that has to happen right at this minute." In this way, she helps me push the huge, potentially ugly scenarios from my head by directing my focus to the small thing I can do right in front of me.

There are people who look out for me in different situations, too. My colleague at work, Lorine, has a special place in my heart for making sure she always has glucose tabs in her purse in case I become hypoglycemic. She knows that I prefer Swedish fish, but she also likes them and is afraid that she would eat them. Despite the fact that I hate those tablets, I love that she carries them with her.

My best friend is an "emotional caregiver" who has gotten me through tense times in my retinologist's waiting room by helping me imagine escaping to beautiful spas and tranquil resorts—all via text message in large fonts. She has also put in endless hours on the phone with me during some frightening battles with complications, listening to my fears and helping me process "my story" until I found the right balance of optimism and realism.

The Real World

It may be a little difficult to get your head around the word "caregiver" in relation to your situation. It was for me.

Use a different word (or no word at all, maybe a phrase, such as "givers of care"), but do not fail to recognize and acknowledge those things that certain people do for us.

Diabetes presents a strange situation to us and the people close to us, because the disability that we experience is often not a constant—it can be very unpredictable as to the type of help we need and when we need it (and how long we need it for). Most of us fall somewhere near the middle of the spectrum. You may be in a situation where you do need help to do most things. More likely, though, you can do many things for yourself, but occasionally need some urgent assistance. Or, the help you need may be a little more involved, in that you need to be driven to most places. Of course, some of us may require more intimate care at times, such as being given a glucagon injection in a hypoglycemic emergency. While it is easy to think that these things are "no big deal," especially for those of us who just need a helping hand occasionally, think back to our prediabetes days. Often a niggling little request from someone or errand that I had to do was enough to throw me off my whole tightly choreographed routine and send me into a tailspin.

So, how do we ensure that those people who help us stay energetic and happy?

Acknowledge their contribution (and burden). Although many people will ask how we, the people with diabetes, are faring during health crises, nobody ever asks the caregiver the same question. They get less attention than usual, even though they are also dealing with increased responsibilities and stress. It is important to remember that these people are not only taking on extra things for us, but they also lost much of our contribution to the "team" for at least a little while, not to mention how hard it often is for them to watch us struggle.

It is crucial that we make an effort to recognize and remind our caregivers (or whatever you want to call them) of everything that they do and how much diabetes has affected their lives, too. Many people in the "helper role" feel strange or guilty thinking of themselves as "burdened," because they compare themselves to us, the people with diabetes, and think about our losses, symptoms and problems. This makes it difficult to face the fact that they need help or support. Remember, these people in our lives are both taking on the things we cannot do, as well as assuming responsibility for extra tasks that come along with helping us.

The Real World

Your caregivers are an important, maybe even crucial, component of your quality of life. Respect them and allow them to have their own feelings and bad days.

Keep them informed. Studies have shown that people in caregiving roles benefit from having as much knowledge as possible about the disease. It is much easier for people to deal with something if they understand something about the "enemy," especially because they do not have the direct physical experience of diabetes. It is important that at least the basic information about the disease comes from other sources besides you. However, you should also share information about your challenges and complications with your caregiver. Show them articles that describe what you are feeling or what you are worried about.

Encourage them to find support. Some caregiver resources include the following:

National Family Caregivers Association (www.thefamilycaregiver.org) works to educate, support and speak up for the more than 50 million Americans who care for loved ones. Their mission is "to empower family caregivers to act on behalf of themselves and their loved ones, and to remove barriers to health and well-being." They do this by linking caregivers to one another in different ways and teaching them to advocate for themselves, including through a volunteer program called Caregiver Community Action Network (CCAN) and through a small online forum. They also have a comprehensive curriculum called "Communicating Effectively with Health Care Professionals," which is comprised of video classes and a series of downloadable forms and articles. They publish a quarterly print and online newsletter called *TAKE CARE!— Self Care for the Family Caregiver*. They can be found online or reached at 800-896-3650.

Well Spouse Association (www.wellspouse.org) is an organization primarily to assist people caring for a disabled spouse. Services include: information about a national network of support groups; facilitating a mentor program and round robin letter writing groups; regional respite weekends and a national conference for caregivers; providing continuing support for members whose spouses have died. Well Spouse Association also publishes a newsletter, called *Mainstay,* and e-newsletter. The Well Spouse Web site contains information around coping and survival skills, including an online forum for spousal caregivers. They can be reached by phone at 800-838-0879.

Today's Caregiver (www.caregiver.com) offers a print and an online version of the *Today's Caregiver* magazine, as well as runs a small forum and an online store with books and videos.

Diversify your team. Even if the majority of extra responsibility will fall to one person, it is much less overwhelming for everyone if there is a backup plan. Ask other people for help, or at least to be on call, besides your spouse or the person who always helps you. I remember once hearing that "If you want someone to be your friend, ask them for help." Many people love to be asked for assistance and would love to do something for you, but they need you to make a specific request.

Also, there are many services that are free of charge or very low cost that can lessen the load in terms of tasks or errands that might fall to other people, such as grocery stores that fill your e-mailed order or pharmacies that deliver.

Make It Better

Do everything in your power to make your caretakers' jobs easier. Give easy-to-follow instructions, find ways to save time and tell them to take some time off when you are having a good day.

Be a team. Again, keep in mind that our helpers not only have the stress of doing extra stuff, they have a front-row seat to the spectacle of our scary bouts with hypoglycemia or limitations introduced by new or worsening complications. It is essential that living with this disease be a team effort. Yes, we are the people with diabetes, but it is often the disease and not us that is setting the bar and making the decisions for us.

Take care of the caregiver. Everyone needs time off. Encourage your helpers to take breaks and do something they enjoy, even if it means that you can't come along. Allow them the freedom to indulge themselves in ways that you can't.

Find humor where you can—and grab it. I have memories that get me through the scary moments. One instance of this occurred after 3 years of my retinologist reassuring me that the retinopathy in my left eye had stabilized, I actually started believing it. The doctor and I spent much of my twice-yearly appointments discussing the hobby we had in common, amateur guitar playing, as I waited for the now-expected "great news" that my retina was still stable. Sure enough, the "great news" continued.

One Wednesday afternoon, a week after my last retinologist appointment, I turned to my co-worker and said calmly, "My eye is bleeding." I found a private place where I could fall apart, then call my doctor and set up an appointment for a few days in the future, as it is impossible to determine the extent of the problem immediately after a hemorrhage. My partner and friends rallied around me, offering constant support, as I nursed fears of "the worst."

The next couple of days, I tried to maintain a sense of "normal" in my life as I looked through the "lava lamp" of the blood in my eye. I had to fake feeling like everything was okay, and my friends were on board with helping me fake it, even though they were worried and walking on eggshells around me. One friend, KR, who sports a shaved head, was peering at me anxiously. I peered back, adjusting my view of him, until I said, "You know, guys, if I position the blood in my left eye just right, it looks like KR's got hair!" The tension was broken and hope flooded in—humor was back and I knew I was going to be okay, regardless of the medical outcome. We all needed to know that.

Bringing Your Diabetes to Work (or Not)

There are many kinds of relationships in the workplace. You have your superiors, your co-workers, the people who work for you and perhaps a whole bunch of other people that keep the place running in some way but have nothing to do with you directly. Your relationships with these various people might be friendly, adversarial, collaborative, or competitive.

Take Charge

Your human resources department may be a confidential place to see about some accommodations at work. The HR people should be able to make things happen without having to tell your manager or co-workers the reason.

It's rather a weird situation, when you think about it. People working full-time often spend more time with the people at their workplace than they do with their spouses or children—certainly this is the case during the week. For many valid reasons, often people with diabetes do not disclose their status to these people that they see every Monday through Friday. However, not mentioning your diabetes doesn't make it go away—in fact, people who choose not to tell anyone are faced with the additional stress of hiding complications and living with a big secret. On the other hand, once you disclose, people are watching you more closely to see how the diabetes is impacting you, including your work. It's a conundrum, no doubt, one that must be worked out by each individual after a number of factors are considered.

In my situation, I take a very matter-of-fact approach to letting people know that I have diabetes, much the same way as I let people know that I am gay—I simply test my blood glucose when I need to with the same lack of fanfare that I mention needing to leave on time to pick up my partner.

However, your situation may be different in terms of what you have shared and what you are comfortable sharing at work. Here are some questions to ask yourself as you think about telling people in the workplace about your diabetes:

Why do I want to disclose my diabetes? Just take the time to think about the answer to this question. Maybe you just are tired of having a secret. Maybe you are feeling that specific complications are interfering with your work and you want to explain this to people.

How do I want to disclose my diabetes? If you are presenting your diabetes as a problem, consider how you could also offer a solution. Maybe there are some accommodations that might help you do your job better that you would like to suggest to your boss as options. Really think about this. Things like a place to rest if you are hypoglycemic or a more flexible work schedule might make a huge difference for you, allowing you to do a better job.

If you are telling co-workers about your diabetes, think about what it will mean to them if you are able to take on less work some days. Consider things from their point of view, then think about what you would want to hear if you were in their place. In many cases, it would be really helpful to prepare people to do stuff that they usually rely on you for with the least amount of effort. Give them the tools they need to work effectively in your absence.

What is the best/worst/most probable result of disclosing my diabetes? We all hope for certain responses when we tell people we have diabetes. In the workplace, it seems like an ideal response would be something along the lines of, "You are so brave for telling us and your exemplary work would never have offered any clue that you had any problems. Of course, we want to do anything to keep you healthy and happy, so please let us know of any accommodations that we can make for you to ensure that you are able to stay with us. Effective immediately, we are cutting your workload by half and giving you a bonus, just for being so wonderful."

You can indulge in a similar little fantasy for a while, but it is important to really think through all the scenarios that you can imagine. That way, you can respond rationally (rather than emotionally) to anything that happens, increasing your odds for the best possible outcome. As someone who has a tendency to blurt things out, and then wonder what the heck just happened, I will tell you that there are some truisms in life, some of which are not pretty, which will apply to your workplace situation:

Information spreads. It just does. You know it as well as I do, people cannot keep secrets. Think about all the "intel" that you have helped travel around the office, whether it was in a gossipy or a matter-of-fact manner. Trust me, your disclosure will not have immunity from this network. Keep this in mind when you tell your office buddy about your diabetes—soon you will probably be watched like a hawk at the morning meetings as people speculate on whether or not you will reach for a donut.

In most situations, a person's first (or second) thought is "how will this affect me?" Even the nicest person will get here eventually. In a workplace, even friendly relationships often have an element of professional give-and-take or teamwork that may be affected by your inability to perform like you used to.

However, people usually want to do the right thing. They do. You can help them to know what the "right thing" is by straight out telling them, "You know what would really help me is if you. . ." If you make people feel like they are part of a "team," they will want to pitch in. Start with things like asking them to make sure to arrange for a break in the middle of a long presentation to clients to have a quick snack or test blood glucose, or that they go over the signs of hypoglycemia with you so that they can help you if needed. Make sure you thank them for their help.

What about disclosing during an interview? Many experts recommend *not* disclosing diabetes status in a job interview, suggesting that you focus instead on the job in question and your abilities to perform the necessary work, even if you will eventually need accommodations.

Brian East, a member of the American Diabetes Association Legal Advocacy Subcommittee and a senior attorney at Advocacy Inc., an Austin, Texas, nonprofit organization that works on behalf of people with disabilities, says, "I always advise people not to lie, and I always advise people to try to avoid answering at the same time. Sometimes that means writing in 'no condition will interfere with me doing this job.'"[1]

Prospective employers are legally not permitted to ask directly about any disease or disability that people may have. However, the fact remains that many people often find themselves in interview situations where someone does ask a question that is illegal or hints around at things. Downright refusing to answer a question or pointing out that a topic that is brought up may be inappropriate will probably not go over well in a job interview. Decide in advance how you are going to handle situations—whether you are going to skirt the issue or be forthright with your diabetes status.

The Bottom Line

It's rather fascinating to watch toddlers get increasingly frustrated when they cannot get people to completely bend to their will. People will say, "It's time for them to learn that they don't control the universe. After all, they are already three." I agree, until I realize that it took me about 40 years to understand that, no matter how hard I try, I cannot control how people are going to behave in a relationship. The person who you thought understood what diabetes is (and what it isn't) may surprise you by joining the chorus of judgment and blame around a new complication, while people that don't even show up on your radar often may come to your rescue.

The Real World

You can't control how people will react to your diabetes, but you can control how and what you tell them. Be thoughtful and goal-driven when talking about your diabetes.

All this is to say that we can only control ourselves. The bitch of it all is, as people with diabetes, we can't even do that all the way. We can't be carefree with what we eat and with our schedules; hypoglycemia may ruin a special evening; a complication may make us needier than we would like to be—all of these things may affect our relationships, especially if we don't address the special challenge that diabetes brings directly through communication with others. The best we can do is to be people who we can be proud of, regardless of the circumstances.

8

Cooperate With Your Emotions

I am aware that there are people out there who truly believe that their diabetes is a blessing, that living with the daily challenges and future unknowns of this disease has brought them to a state of grace.

I am *absolutely* not one of them.

Having gotten that out of the way, let me tell you how I really feel about the whole thing. Diabetes can be sneaky and insidious. It is like living with a time bomb. Just when I get comfortable with my routine and forget about my diabetes for a little while, a little "challenge" like hypoglycemia knocks me off my feet for a short time. Human nature (or my nature) being what it is, 15 or 20 minutes later when I am feeling better, the moment is all but forgotten.

However, diabetes does not tolerate denial or complacency and will occasionally remind me of that in a more dramatic way. *Wham*! A blood vessel in my eye ruptures. My heart rate accelerates in a scary way. My stomach decides to stop digesting.

These things have happened enough times that even when I am coasting along in reasonably good health, I am very aware of how vulnerable my body is and how quickly my fragile sense of calm well-being can disappear.

You can't escape your emotions—living with this disease and making choices about how to proceed in your life with diabetes is fraught with feelings. As you try to look at statistics and "likelihoods" when making decisions about treatments or future plans, your emotions may pull you away from looking at things scientifically and acting rationally. You will learn that not only is it okay to act in accord with emotions, it is also desirable to give your feelings "a vote" in important matters, or underlying worry and stress will always be present. It is also crucial to understand when negative feelings become destructive and need to be addressed (and how to do it).

Honor Your Feelings, but Stop When You Are Done

It seems like every time negative emotions are discussed in regard to diabetes, it is by "experts" who mention feelings like anger, sadness and self-pity as "impediments to adherence." In other words, they worry about us feeling crappy because this may make us less likely to check our blood glucose, follow our food plans, or take our meds as prescribed. It is almost as if, upon diagnosis, we became puzzled to figure out what parts of ourselves contribute to "good" glucose control, and which aspects of our actions and personalities stand in the way of that goal of physicians and researchers alike. However, we all remain people after our diagnosis, and being a human brings with it emotions, some of them negative.

Take Charge

Be angry, be sad, be afraid, be lonely—then stop. Repeat when necessary. Just don't forget to stop.

So, as a person actually living with diabetes, I'll offer up an account of what these emotions feel like to me. I am sure that your experience with all of them is different, but equally valid. In my opinion, "speaking the truth" about these often-ugly feelings helps them do their good work of helping us process undesirable things, which are often beyond our control, but it also helps limit their potential for destruction.

Anger

My anger mostly comes when this disease hurts. It never hurts in a vacuum; others are always involved.

Years ago, an unusual case of retinopathy brought me to the point of legal blindness, which helped me make the decision to have vitrectomy performed. All went smoothly—vision was restored, but I was left looking terrible and in desperate need of cheering up. I sought out the very people who were sure to lift my spirits: my young niece and nephew, whom I adore. I couldn't wait to see them and bask in their company. However, my heart broke and anger at my diabetes overwhelmed me at the reaction of these enthusiastic children when they saw Aunt Lynn. My nephew hugged me gingerly and quickly backed away, while his sister hid and cried because I was hurt.

Although I am frequently frustrated at what diabetes does to me and the limits that it has imposed, most of my true anger has come from the moments where my diabetes has hurt others, such as my mom having to worry about two kids with type 1 diabetes at a time when few tools were available, and it was far more dangerous; the occasions when I have scared my partner with a hypoglycemic free fall in the middle of the night; or threat of the unknown future implications of some of my more challenging complications.

The Real World

Your anger is waiting, looking for an excuse to come out. Don't confuse the excuse with the real source—in many cases, your diabetes.

Other people may find themselves outwardly directing the anger at what is happening inside their body. Although it is hard to control sometimes, realize that anger is often expressed as irritability or sarcasm directed at those that happen to just be standing in the way of it. Try not to lash out at those innocent bystanders. It can also come out at unexpected times in a completely overblown reaction to something small. In her insightful and articulate book, *Life Disrupted: Getting Real About Chronic Illness in Your Twenties and Thirties*, Laurie Edwards recounts an incident in which she had a self-described "meltdown" over the wrong salad dressing being included with a dinner delivery order. She talks about weeping inconsolably after flinging the salad in the trash can, and finding it difficult to articulate why the "crappy Greek dressing symbolized all the tiny little aggravations that had accumulate over the years."

Fear and Anxiety

I try to keep my anxiety at bay by actively working to control my blood glucose through discipline and strong education about and effort around my treatment plans. After all, I will assure myself, I am power-ful against this disease, and surely there is nothing to be afraid of.

Then a new symptom, real or imagined, unlocks the mental box containing all of the worst-case scenario visions of the future with some new physical limitation. My fear screams at me when a shadow crosses my vision. Surely, this must be a hemorrhage. Long after the appointment where the retinologist assures me that I am fine and that everything in my eye is stable, the anxiety lingers. For the rest of the day, fear and anxiety are still so acute that I am prevented from hearing the good news.

Don't Panic

Diabetes is scary, it is. Make it less scary by turning unknowns into knowns and uncontrollables into controllables whenever you can.

Much fear comes from uncertainty, from being unable to control the future. When you are in the midst of being afraid, it doesn't help to recognize the fact that for most people, living with diabetes or not, "control" is an illusion anyway. Any of us could have our lives turned upside down by a recession in which we experience financial losses, natural disasters, and one of our family members being diagnosed with a health problem. Clearly, those of us with diabetes and our family members do live with a specific kind of uncertainty and must be able to respond, rather than freezing up, making it necessary to find the bal-ance between living in abject fear of disease progression and ignoring real changes that need attention.

If fear and anxiety stemming from uncertainty last for too long, people may do harmful and impulsive things to try and gain control. They may begin to defy their treatment plan without telling their doctor and turn to potentially dangerous complementary and alterna-tive medicine approaches. They may also make drastic changes to their lives, such as moving, leaving relationships or solidifying unhealthy ones, or quitting jobs. Although very difficult to do while in the grasp of fear, it is crucial to distinguish between things that can be controlled and those that cannot. We can then strategize how to man-age the things that we can influence and adapt to the things beyond our immediate control.

I have an image that I use to keep myself sane when I feel like I am sitting on a time bomb of complications, as I often do, never knowing when something will explode and disrupt my life, despite the efforts that I am constantly making to manage my blood glucose. Although I can get by most days dealing with those things that I have to deal with and not letting fear of bigger complications take over, sometimes it is too much and I get scared. I have found that I am too much of a realist to live in denial (besides, diabetes will usually remind me of its presence in an unpleasant way if I do this for too long).

I therefore have come up with the idea of "the shelf." The shelf is where I keep my box of fears and issues. This image works out great for me, as it allows me to take out these fears and examine them and let them deflate a little, then I imagine placing them back in the box and shutting the lid. I make sure that I really visualize myself putting the box back on the shelf, so that I don't have to carry this box—this burden—with me as I go through my days.

Sadness

Sadness feels rather passive to me. I think, at least for me, that it comes along with being emotionally fatigued over it. I want a break and know I am not going to get one.

For other people with diabetes, sadness has different, more specific roots. Clearly, any complication that imposes physical limits on us brings sadness to us and to our loved ones. However, there are other things that we have lost, but that we may feel are trivial. These things can make us sad, as well as feel petty. Let's face it; it *is* sad that you can no longer be carefree about what you eat and when you sleep. It *is* sad that other women can enjoy their pregnancies, focusing on nursery colors and maternity fashion, while you have to monitor blood glucose 10 times a day and think about every bite you eat. It *is* sad that your mom starts every conversation with "how are your numbers?" rather than asking about your new job. These things are not silly. They are losses and you are allowed to grieve them. You are allowed to be sad.

A special note about sadness: If you have diabetes and feel very sad or have no interest in things around you, you need to seek help—especially if you have had these feelings for 2 weeks or more and they are interfering with your daily life. Depression is very common in people with diabetes. It is nothing to be embarrassed about, it is not your fault and it can be treated. If not addressed, it is shown to contribute to poor outcomes as people may begin to neglect themselves and let their treatment regimen lapse. Get help.

Loneliness

You are right. *They* don't understand. However, you don't really need them to. Invisible symptoms are very difficult for others to comprehend, and much of my loneliness comes from people actually trying to connect by relating discomforts or problems that they have to my diabetes, by offering up statements to the effect of, "Oh, I know what you are going through. I have to watch what I eat, too." Maybe even worse is when people try to make me feel better in a patronizing way—"You're doing great for someone with diabetes. If you have to monitor yourself that closely, it's amazing that you do anything else." These kind of statement only serve to make me feel "other" in a particularly isolating way.

Make It Better

Talk to people who *do* understand you, and the full range of your emotions about having diabetes. Make an effort to cultivate friends who also have diabetes but who share your approach to living with the disease.

We often avoid contact with others when we are feeling our worst, most affected by our symptoms, having the hardest time emotionally, are afraid to burden people or be pitied. However, this is precisely when we need contact the most. Years ago, my grandmother gave me an article that contained a line I remember to this day—"surround yourself with people that offer you hope."

Honor Your Negative Emotions, Then Stop

People have told me that I am courageous. That I am a survivor. I know they mean well, but really, what choice is there? The alternative to continuing to try is to give up, which is one thing when you are training for a fun run, but has entirely different implications when you have type 1 diabetes. I don't always feel brave and I don't always feel happy. Sometimes I am very scared and I am often just over it all. I bet many, if not most, of us feel this way occasionally.

How can we interact these emotions in a way that we get "what we need" from them, but still are able to escape? In my opinion, it is a good thing to occasionally wallow in these emotions. I have learned through the challenges that I have faced that I need to sit in the shitty feelings before I can move past them. I need to feel the "not fair" and the "what next" and the "this sucks" moments deeply and fully, to process them and chew them up and digest them. Then I make a plan.

Plans can differ, but need to be action oriented, as "planning to be happier" usually doesn't get us very far. I suggest listing everything that you might want to do to fight back against this disease (or a certain aspect of it), which may include: tracking your symptoms, getting a second opinion, conducting a little research to see what your options are, talking to people—whatever it takes to make you feel like you are participating, to make you feel like you are acting, rather than reacting to your circumstances.

For me, making a plan gives me hope. And, in this situation, hope is the ladder that I use to climb up out of the swamp of negative emotions. Hope is what makes me the brave person, the survivor, that people believe I am.

Dabble in Benefit-finding

Benefit-finding is basically looking for positive results of an adverse thing in one's life: "every cloud has a silver lining," "always look on the bright side," stuff like that. When it comes to benefit-finding and diabetes, there seem to be two types of people with diabetes: those who say their diabetes has been a blessing and those who get violent upon hearing such a statement. Interestingly, research shows that people who are able to see some positive aspects of having diabetes had improved relationships, more appreciation for life, and deepened spirituality. These people also tended to reevaluate priorities, focus more on their families, and make positive lifestyle changes.

You may not be ready to wholeheartedly embrace the idea that diabetes is a net positive in your life. In fact, if you are like me, at this very moment you may be on the verge of screaming, "Diabetes is no friggin' blessing and don't you dare say anything else stupid like 'at least it's not cancer!' " However, agree as we may that diabetes is not a special gift that has been bestowed upon us, even I can concede that diabetes has led me to make some positive choices. I take care of myself. I exercise and stay in good shape. I have a career that I like and I speak my mind at work.

The Real World

Be fair to your diabetes. Don't blame your diabetes for being bad at math (if you were never good at it); don't blame your diabetes for marital problems (especially those that would be there anyway). Be fair to your diabetes and determine what suffering it is causing and what suffering isn't its fault.

I guess the point here is to not blame the diabetes for all that is not perfect in your life and, in the same vein, give the diabetes credit where it is due. All that might not outweigh the negative aspects of having diabetes and all the crappy complications that are part of the package, but thinking about it in this way may help release some of the anger if you let it.

The Bottom Line

We did not ask for diabetes; none of us did. Yet, here we are, many of us forced to strategically plan things that other people do without a thought, the things of life—eating, working, playing, sleeping, waking—all of it becomes part of the diabetes equation on some level. This gets tiring.

When I was experiencing a rapid heart rate (as a symptom of my cardiac autonomic neuropathy), I remember sitting on my deck at night. I was consumed by fear and anger, with the dramatic racing of my heart providing the fuel for these feelings. This time in my life, battling this complication, brought home more than ever the overwhelming knowledge that I can't get away from my diabetes—it comes with me and will be with me for the rest of my life. Even my closest people, those who care about me and worry about me the most, can escape it for a while. I can't and that is a lonely, lonely feeling.

This does not mean that we should avoid being sad or angry, as if this is even possible. Sometimes we need to sit down and visit with these emotions. Without looking in the *Diagnostic and Statistical Manual of Mental Disorders, Fourth Edition* (*DSM-IV*), I don't know how angry is "too angry"—is it okay to be mad, but not furious, for instance—or the exact length of time that someone can feel sorry for themselves or anxious before they cross a line. Despite how it might seem at times, I don't think that most of us even get close to being diagnosable as we explore the "dark side." I think it is a necessary part of coping with this disease.

However, eventually we must find our way out. I guess everyone has a different strategy. I focus on making my plan to take action against that which was making me scared or sad. Knowing that I have a list of things that I can actually do—focusing on the process, not the outcome—gives me hope. Hope is what opens the drapes wide and lets the light in.

9

Get "in the Mix"

As people living with diabetes, many of our struggles are our own and our situations are unique. However, there are many people living with diabetes out there, experiencing similar fears, challenges, and successes. We watch for new research and treatment developments. We weather disappointments around failed trials or adverse events at the same time. Connecting to others with diabetes can open up new sources of inspiration and understanding. We can learn from others' trials, changing our lives for the better.

Are Self-help Groups for You?

Some people love self-help or support groups, and others really just don't like the whole idea. I have to admit here that I am not a huge fan of participating in support groups for myself, because I have worked hard to construct a support system of friends and family members that know what I need and when I need it in terms of support. However, too many people with diabetes feel guilty and perceive that others are blaming them for their diabetes and any related complications. They feel that they are being judged, rather than supported, by those close to them. For these people, support groups can be invaluable, empowering people and dispelling feelings of shame so that they can take action to care for themselves.

Self-help groups have become an integral part of treatment for emotional issues, behavior problems, mental health problems, and for dealing with stressful situations. Many people find that support groups are an invaluable resource for recovery and for empowerment. In the ideal situation, a support group is a group of people who deeply understand each other and can offer practical advice and emotional reinforcement—from the names of good doctors (and those to avoid) to a shoulder to cry on.

Let's start with talking about what self-help groups are—in general, these are groups of people with a similar problem or health condition that come together on a voluntary basis to get support from each other. The idea is that the participants can gain from one another's experiences dealing with the same problems, offering practical advice and strategies, as well as emotional support. Participants can discuss things that only others with diabetes could understand and can feel "safe" when revealing their emotions around this disease. The ultimate desired result of participation in such a group would be renewed self-confidence in dealing with diabetes, stemming from emotional support and practical directions to take.

In my opinion, one of the reasons that many of us do not find support groups to be "right" for us is that diabetes affects such a diverse group of people and the challenges of controlling blood glucose and complications differ drastically among individuals. A 12-step program is so very effective for some people because, even though all participants are different, they are focused on one goal (abstaining from alcohol, gambling or drugs, or confronting another problem) using a very specific formula. Thus, all the participants speak a "common language," even though they might be in different stages of recovery or relapse.

The Real World

Diabetes is a disease with diversity. There are various complications and two (main) types of diabetes, all with different degrees of severity in each individual. Add to that the unique financial and social situations of each individual and you end up with quite a few differences between two people with diabetes.

Although it may work in some cases, a group that is formed around the kernel of diabetes as the common factor may just be too diverse to work. You could end up with a teenager newly diagnosed with type 1 diabetes trying to figure out how to fit in at school with her new identity; a 67-year-old woman who has been threatened by her doctor to "get serious" about lifestyle changes or she may be facing "the needle" (and has no idea where to start or what to do); a middle-aged man with type 2 diabetes contemplating bariatric surgery; and someone who was diagnosed as prediabetic and wants to learn more.

Luckily, many people are starting to recognize this and support groups are starting to differentiate across different lines. For instance, in New York City, one can find Sugar, a support group for LGBT (lesbian, gay, bisexual, transgender) people with diabetes, run by ACT1 Diabetes (**www.act1diabetes.org**). The Joslin Diabetes Center (**www.jolslin.org**) has a Latino Support Group, conducted entirely in Spanish, in which "participants find comfort in the commonality of diabetes, their language, and the immigrant experience."

Make It Better

Don't overlook similarities and what connects you with others amid diabetes differences.

However, if you can't find a group that is just right for you, a place where you feel like you are among supportive friends, where you can let your true self shine, there are plenty of ways to engage with other people with diabetes. It is important to do this for yourself—whether you connect with them virtually or by telephone, or even by forming your own group, the benefits are worth doing a little digging and extra work. We'll talk about some of the other ways that people with diabetes maintain contact with each other a little later in the chapter.

Rules of Engagement

Support groups can be great. However, this might be a different type of social situation than you are used to. They are basically comprised of strangers (in the beginning) who come together to share pretty personal stuff: things that they may not even tell their families or friends. These strangers may also be seeking emotional support that they are not getting from loved ones. Because many "normal" steps in a typical getting-to-know-each-other social process get skipped, it may be wise to strategize the best way to go about things to make sure that you get what you want and need out of these accelerated "insta-friend" situations.

Think About What You Want From a Support Group

People come to support groups for different reasons. Some come seeking emotional support because they are lonely and feel isolated, living in a world of healthy people who don't "get it." Others are on a mission to find out specific information about how to deal with specific complications, tips for using their insulin pumps, or to get a recommendation for a good endocrinologist. Many are just at a loss and don't know where to go. Then there are some people that just want to be able to be themselves in a crowd that understands, discusses potentially embarrassing problems freely, and even have a couple of much-needed laughs that people without diabetes may find macabre or inappropriate.

Get Help

Virtual support includes online chat rooms, discussion groups, forums, and just simple e-mail exchanges that you find value in.

Before you head into a social situation, whether an in-person support group or a virtual meeting place, put some thought into what you want to get out of the group. This will help you find the right forum for you, as you can evaluate different settings and tones of groups easily when you have a personal standard by which you are measuring it. This is not to say that you won't find a group of people that you end up joining and loving, but which has nothing to do with your original "wish list," but it does mean that you might be able to avoid some disappointment by evaluating things objectively from the outset. For example, if you are seeking support and advice about how to deal with starting insulin injections, a group called *Pump Perspectives* is probably not an exact fit for your specific need, although you may share some of their ideals and wishes and eventually make this your group of choice.

Think About Who You Want to Be in a Support Group

Take Charge

One of the easiest ways to join a group is to meet a member beforehand for coffee (or even a phone call) and have that person introduce you to the group. That way you get a chance to ask questions before attending to see if the group is a good fit, and you already know someone when you arrive. It makes a huge difference.

Yes, we are all people with diabetes. However, in most cases, that is not enough of a common thread to ensure that you will automatically click with a particular group right off the bat. Ideally, you will eventually find a group where you can let it all hang out. Until you are comfortable, however, take some time and watch the dynamics of different groups to find your point of entry and face that you would like to present. For instance, if you are in a support group for newly diagnosed people who are working through their initial feelings about having diabetes and struggling with treatment decisions, you may not want to start your introduction by saying things like "I hate listening to crybabies who are afraid to give themselves injections."

The Real World

Don't feel bad about "shopping" different support groups. You need to find a group that is a good fit for you. If you choose not to be in a group, it is not a judgment on the group, it just means that that group was not right for you at this time in your life.

Think What Kind of Relationships You Want in a Support Group

To say it is wise to be strategic to get what you need out of a support group may sound calculated and manipulative, but it does not hurt to think about things before you jump in and relationships get established. If you really just want to hear about how others are coping with their anger or sadness, realize that if you announce that you are considering participating in a stem cell clinical trial, that will become a focus of attention, rather than your emotional needs.

Do Your Best

As with anything else, you have to give something to get something. Be prepared to offer emotional and other types of support to fellow group members.

Rules to Get the Most Out of a Group

> *Rule 1: Be a good listener.* This might mean biting your tongue if someone says something that you think is

wrong or forcing yourself to sit through a really long boring story when you have an excellent anecdote that is much more appropriate to the situation and could even bring a couple of laughs. You will get your turn to talk.

Rule 2: Find out the expectations of the group. If the group members all commit to come on a regular basis and actively participate each time, make sure that you want to do that. Otherwise, you could disrupt the flow and end up not fitting in well.

Rule 3: Be respectful of others. This goes beyond general manners of not laughing at someone or not interrupting when it comes to participating in a diabetes support group. You must remember that we are all on a different journey and that diabetes has a different impact on all of us, physically, mentally and emotionally. Never compare your situation to others'—although someone's mild hypoglycemia experience may seem trivial in comparison to your recent ketoacidosis crisis when you had the flu, other people's fears and discomforts are surely a big deal to them. None of us pictured ourselves dealing with any of the crap that diabetes throws our way, and none of us are "lucky" that we "only" have certain symptoms.

Finding a Support Group

Your doctor may know about a support group in your area, and certainly, a certified diabetes educator (CDE) would have a couple of recommendations for you. You could also enter "diabetes support group" and the name of your city into Google or another search engine for ideas. Here are a couple of resources to check out during your search:

TuDiabetes.org allows people to post about different support groups and get-togethers in their state. The neat thing about this site is that people write in to mention all sorts of things that are going on in their area, including classes, expos, and fund-raising events. I have also seen several people in an area form a "group" of their own after meeting on this site and arranging to get together in person. To see what is going on in your state, go to www.tudiabetes.org, select "Groups" from the menu bar at the top of the page, click on "USA Groups" and your state when the map of the United States pops up.

Defeat Diabetes Foundation has a list of "Diabetes Support Groups and Education Programs" listed by state. Get there by going to **www.defeatdiabetes.org**, then clicking on "Support Groups" under the "Self-Management" tab on the top menu. The vast majority of listings are of various education programs and centers affiliated with hospitals and clinics—however, the staff at one of these places can probably give you the names of several support groups in your area, including ones affiliated with their program.

Depending on several factors, such as the size of your city and the activity level of the diabetes community there, there may be several groups to choose from. For instance, a large city may have specific groups for all sorts of different people with diabetes with different interests and formats. On the other hand, if you live in a smaller city or town, you may only find one or two groups that are convenient to you. Make sure that you call the coordinator to find out if this group is right for you. Some groups welcome families and friends, while others are just for people living with diabetes. Some are more like classes with lectures on specific topics, some groups meet for lunch, some have speakers come in, and some are to provide an understanding and supportive environment for any type of discussion that may arise.

Make It Better

If someone is helpful or you would like to know someone better from your support group, have lunch with them or give them a call. These interactions outside the group setting can be very valuable.

Meet the Diabetes Community From the Comfort of Your Own Home

There are lots of reasons that many of us like to interact with other people with diabetes from home. Maybe there is no support group within a convenient distance from your home or maybe it is difficult for you to get out for one reason or another. Perhaps you are not ready to sit in a room with other people with diabetes in an unstructured support atmosphere and you prefer discussing very specific topics with anonymous people. Regardless of your reasons, topics of interest, and style of communication, there is a whole world of virtual "friends" waiting to meet you and offer, as well as receive, much-needed support, advice, and new ideas.

Take Charge

The Internet can be great, but you do need to balance your "screen time" with other activities. Be a bit goal oriented, set time limits, and don't stay on the computer so long that you feel weird rejoining real life.

Health researchers have looked into why people used online support sites and found that the people that were the most active on these sites loved things like convenience and access to information, but they also liked the ability to ask advice and the lack of embarrassment when dealing with personal issues. Studies found that many people perceive improvements in quality of life and report that their health complaints or symptoms are less severe since they joined the site. However, there are some health professionals that point to evidence that too much time in the virtual world can lead to isolation and depression, especially if it is at the expense of socializing with friends.

Special Rules for Participating in an Online Group to Get the Most Out of It

Rule 1: Open up. You are anonymous when online, so you can be more open and free with your opinions and feelings. Use this situation wisely—express feelings that you have been keeping bottled up, share embarrassing experiences, let out your frustrations.

Rule 2: Pause a moment. However, think before you type and reread posts before you send them to ensure that you are not inadvertently offending someone and that you are communicating what you intend to.

Rule 3: Guard your identity. Be cautious, even paranoid, about sharing personal information—don't post telephone numbers and don't use e-mail addresses comprised of your full name.

The Real World

When a jerk is harassing you in a forum (and there will be at least one), my favorite strategy is to thank them. Not only is it classy, but it takes all the fun out of tormenting you, which usually results in the person leaving you alone. Just something, slightly tongue-in-cheek, like "Thank you so much for your thoughtful insights," can take the air out of anyone's mean sails.

Rule 4: Cool down. Don't respond immediately to a post or message that has offended or angered you. Reread it a couple of times and realize that people often have a difficult time communicating accurately in writing, or may not understand "netiquette," such as ALL CAPS MEANS THAT YOU ARE SHOUTING. Even if you do decide that the poster has truly intended to tell you that you are stupid, for example if they type, "I cannot believe how very stupid you are," think before you answer. Drowning a mean person in virtual honey often serves one better than going on the attack, as others feel free to participate in the discussion and come to the defense of the "victim" of the nastiness.

Take Charge

If you find you are wasting precious energy worried about how people responded to your message or trying to think up ways to change someone's mind in a debate, it may be time to leave that forum. Life is too short to bring negative energy from the Internet into it.

Forums and Message Boards

A forum is an interesting way to "talk" to other people with diabetes and find answers to specific questions. There are many forums out there for people with diabetes, but I am going to mention a couple to get you started, depending on what type of information or virtual environment you are looking for:

TuDiabetes.org is "a community of people touched by diabetes" and is run by the Diabetes Hands Foundation. It runs forums for people with all types of diabetes, including prediabetes. I love that it has a "search" feature to zero in on a discussion that may be of interest to you (not all forums have this feature). If you are checking out this forum for the first time, I recommend that you go to the dropdown menu on the right that says "View" and choose "Categories" to find your peeps. DiabetesDaily.com and DiabeticConnect.com also have forums for people with all types of diabetes. You may get different "vibes" from different forums, so it is worth checking out a couple.

Juvenation.org is an online community for people with type 1 diabetes, which is run by the Juvenile Diabetes Research Foundation. Scroll down to "Discussions" on the forum page to see the main topic areas that are discussed.

DiabetesSisters.org is all about women's issues. This is a very pretty site, with the bonus of some fun features. One cool thing here is the "Diabetes Buddy Program" that can match you with someone who has similar interests and goals as you, so that you can communicate and support each other for a 6-week period. There is also a free reminder program (to check glucose, to take meds, to whatever) that you can use. DiabetesSisters puts on a yearly Weekend for Women Conference for women living with diabetes.

Make It Better

Make a pledge to try to reach out to others a couple of different ways. Find others with diabetes. Make a connection.

Blog it. It has been shown that writing about traumatic experiences actually has healing properties. I don't know if the theory applies to the extent that a heartfelt pouring out of emotions about the challenges of diabetes onto your computer screen would make any difference in your A1c results, but it might be just the catharsis that you need to get through a rough patch. "Blog" is short for "Web log" and is a loose term for a site that is maintained with regular entries of personal essays, news, or other kinds of commentary. There are many, many people with diabetes out there who maintain blogs. Check out The Diabetes Resource (**www.thediabetesresource.com**) and look for "Diabetes

Bloggers" under the "Directory" tab to find a listing of over 270 blogs. You will find something for everyone here, whether you have type 1 diabetes, type 2, LADA, or have a child with diabetes. By messing around on the site a little and visiting other blogs, you will see the opportunity to contribute to someone's blog or even create your own. The majority of blogs have a space for people to comment, which is often a way of starting a conversation around the topic covered in a specific blog post.

The following are some blogs that I think deserve special mention:

Managing the Sweetness Within (www.thesweetnesswithin.blogspot.com). A well-written, insightful blog by a woman who successfully navigated a pregnancy with type 1 diabetes. She chronicles the details of not just the months of carrying a baby, but the whole process, including fun (yet graphic) details of her IVF attempts and breastfeeding.

diaTribe (www.diatribe.us). Actually more of an online "newsletter" than a blog, this site focuses entirely on "research and product news for people with diabetes." This is an impressive site with contributions from articulate people with strong opinions about diabetes and what is being done in the world of research and tangible progress in treatments for diabetes.

Living with Diabetes and Lapband (www.kweaver.org/blog). This blog is written by a woman with type 2 diabetes who had lapband surgery. According to the author, Kathleen Weaver, this is the oldest diabetes blog there is, dating back to February 28, 2003. This blog truly gives insight into a life with type 2 diabetes, before and after lapband surgery: It is warm, human, and incredibly honest, sparing no details of forgotten medications, glucose readings and the emotions that go with them, and stresses from a real life with diabetes and the solutions that worked at that moment.

Facebook and other social networking. You can also consider creating and maintaining a page on Facebook (**www.facebook.com**), which gives you a little more control over what parts of your site people have access to. Lots of big organizations and publications have Facebook pages addressing diabetes, as well as hundreds of individuals who focus on different health concerns and advocacy issues around diabetes. There are pages that give you info to help you manage your diabetes, pages dedicated to fund raising for a specific organization, pages for "pumpers," pages by people who have had lapband surgery— you name it, you will find a topic close to your heart here. Visit a couple of these pages (create a page in Facebook, then enter "diabetes" in the search box) to get an idea of the diversity of what is out there and how you may want to organize your page.

The Bottom Line

There is no question about it. Diabetes is a very lonely disease, even if we are surrounded by helpful and understanding people who love us. There are no words to describe how overwhelming the idea of "doing diabetes" for the rest of our lives can become at times, and we may end up self-editing everything that we say or do in order not to appear whiny or needy or anything but perfectly fine to those around us.

Get Help

There are lots of reasons to connect with other people with diabetes, but one of the best reasons is to gain a little bit of perspective. We are not alone; others have gone before us, and we will get through it (somehow).

It seems that for many of us, meeting other people with diabetes, whether in person or virtually, would be like having a cozy little clubhouse where we were exclusive members.

What we need to remember is that there are others suffering alone out there, and what we really need to do is get together and be able to laugh about things that might otherwise make us cry, and cry about things that no one else would understand.

10

Make Things Better

For those of us living with diabetes, the demands can be incessant and the worries always hover in the back of our minds. We learn to deal with our inner demons and keep our moods uplifted. However, every so often—maybe rarely for some, much more often for others—there comes a moment when we are made to understand that there is something that we can't do because we have diabetes and the needs that go along with it. Maybe we are reprimanded at work for taking a break to check our blood glucose. Maybe you are told that you are not "healthy enough" to be on a sports team. Maybe you are not given the chance for a make up exam when you missed the test because of hypoglycemia.

Some of these things we can tolerate. However, at some point, there just has to be a *no*, maybe even a *NO!* It may be a seemingly insignificant moment that changes your views on life and what is right for you—an overheard joke about a celebrity's diabetes, a doctor who accuses you of not following orders because you haven't lost weight on his schedule, or an argument with your insurance company over paying for a prescribed treatment. Or, you may have a bigger epiphany arising from a crisis that alters your outlook, while the world kept on about business as usual.

Make It Better

If we all agree to make things better whenever we can, our worlds—both individually and as a member of the community of people with diabetes—will be slowly, but steadily, improving.

Being your own advocate means standing up for yourself by understanding your rights and fighting for them. It means figuring out what is right for you or what you need, then making sure that you get it. To be your own best advocate, you may have to turn your preconceived ideas of authority upside down. You have to remember that you are the expert in what you need, and eliminate notions that others know better, that the system is impossible to navigate or that things are too hard to change.

You can change from a passive patient to an active advocate for your own health care and your rights as a person living with diabetes. The things that will make you an active advocate are simple, but not easy for everyone to do. You will have to examine personal assumptions about authority figures and health care that are still deeply ingrained in the culture. You will learn that you can, indeed, be your own advocate.

Universal Approaches to Advocacy, or How to Get What You Want

Many people associate advocacy with hand-lettered signs and lots of screaming about volatile issues, which get covered on the evening news, biased toward one extreme position or another. However, advocacy is simply the act of speaking up in an attempt to change things for the better, whether it is just for yourself in a particular situation or for a larger group.

Regardless if you are trying to get something done that you need or trying to tackle a problem for the greater good, there are some keys to increasing your chances of success.

Principle 1: Define your problem precisely and be very specific about what you want to change.

Unfortunately, when we get upset and emotional about something, many of us also tend to get less articulate about what the problem is. Putting your head in your hands and weeping to the doctor that you "just need a break from diabetes" will not tell him or her what he or she needs to fix. If you let the doctor know more specifically that you are overwhelmed by trying to figure out food counts or that you got scared when you were hypoglycemic earlier that morning, this gives the doctor a good starting place to figure out what the next steps might be.

> ### Take Charge
>
> No one can help you make a difference unless you know what you want. Avoid wasting your (and others') time by just venting or expressing the injustice of things. Have a clearly defined goal when you seek change.

Principle 2: Have a well-researched solution to offer.

In your desire to make something in your life better, you may get emotional and make assumptions that people know what to do to help you. For instance, you may decide that your job is too physically demanding, even though you love it. Going to your boss and crying, "it's just too hard, I can't keep up, but please don't fire me," does not give your boss much to work with and puts him or her in an awkward situation. However, outlining different ideas for adjusting your schedule, allowing you to work from home on specific projects, or making modifications to your work space or the way that you do things shows that the job means something to you and that you want to work something out.

> ### Know Your Stuff
>
> Knowing the options will prevent you from making mistakes or pursuing the wrong path. A bit of research before seeking a solution can save time, effort, and money.

Likewise, telling your doctor in a moment of frustration that you *cannot stand* injecting insulin anymore and giving the simple directive to "fix this" sends the message that this is your priority above all else. Your doctor may skip trying to troubleshoot and go straight for something like an insulin pump in an attempt to relieve your distress. However, you may be unprepared for various aspects of the pump that you have not thought through. Minor consequences of not communicating precisely might include wasting time that could have been used to solve your problem with more conservative measures or, more dramatically, you may end up taking actions that you end up regretting.

Principle 3: Figure out who can solve your problem, then focus on that specific decision maker.

In some cases it probably *seems* very clear whom you are trying to influence and who has access to what you need to make things better for yourself. When you are trying to deal with a symptom medically, a logical "target" seems to be your doctor. When you have decided that adjusting your work schedule to allow for "flex time" would help you cope with your fatigue or other symptoms of complications, you would no doubt start by talking to your immediate supervisor.

However, when you are going after what you want, make sure you take the time and think things through all the way. Remember, most people operate within a hierarchical structure and it might take a couple of tries and some patience to find out who holds the keys to resolving your problem. For instance, your doctor might need to get a procedure preapproved from your insurance company before proceeding and your immediate supervisor will probably need to get approval from someone higher up in the company before granting your request.

Do Your Best

Sure, we are angry, but when advocating for change, we need to make allies, not enemies. Evoke sympathy and help people help us.

Be patient as you climb up the ladder in trying to fix your issue. It helps to put yourself in the place of the person you are dealing with at each step and realize that most people really just don't want to get in trouble and want to do things with the least amount of stress to themselves as possible. Think back to times that you may have gotten upset about things and attacked the first person that had to tell you bad news—you may have ended up screaming at the customer service representative at your phone company for an overcharge, it may have been that the line at airport security was too long and you missed your plane so you let loose on the guy checking identification and boarding passes, it may be that your insurance company denied payment for a medication and you gave the pharmacist an earful about it. Not only were these people most likely not able to help solve your problem, you probably alienated someone who might have been helpful in getting you in front of the right person or finding an alternative solution. I know I have learned this lesson the "hard way," and probably not for the last time, although I do my best to fight the urge to take out my frustration on the first person standing in my way.

Principle 4: Be assertive and confident, not aggressive and combatant, in your communications.

Although advocacy is fighting to get what you want, the method behind the "fight" might not look like any fight you've ever seen (or fought). Standing up for yourself is an act of preserving and pursuing dignity— as such, it should be done in a dignified manner.

People who are assertive and confident seem to be in control— they are folks who are going to get what they want because it is right and because it is how the world should work. People listen to those individuals who can present their views in a way that makes everything they say come across as objective fact, thus it is more likely that people will work to help them.

To come across as authoritative, but likeable, a couple of things need to be kept in mind. Most importantly, stay calm and cool. Never insult or threaten the other person. That makes people focus on themselves (and their feelings of anger at you), while taking their attention away from your problem. It is important to stick to the topic that you are discussing and not let emotions take you into other territory of other unrelated issues. You can ask the other person if you are communicating clearly (this is kind of a trick to reset him or her and make sure that the person is getting the message)—I often say something like, "You know, I appreciate your time. This is so important to me that I just want to make sure that my emotions are not interfering with what I want to say. Have you understood what I said so far, or have I left out something?" Listen carefully when the other person talks. Ask the other person to clarify his or her point or repeat important information.

Principle 5: Keep notes and track your progress.

Do Your Best

If you don't write it down and can't remember important details, it is like it never happened.

Whether you are talking to your endocrinologist, your insurance company, or your lawyer, it is important to be able to present your facts. Consider these two exchanges:

"Hi, I hope you can help me out. On November 2nd of this year, I spoke with Mary Cramer in customer service about the refusal of payment for my laser photocoagulation that I received on October 10th. She told me that it was a matter of a problem with the form submitted by my retinologist's office, in that it did not reflect that this procedure was a continuation of the preapproved one that was started the day before, but had to be stopped because the doctor was called away on an emergency. I called my retinologist's office the same day that I spoke with Ms. Cramer and explained the situation. They pulled up the record and saw their error, which they promised to rectify that same day and resubmit the form by fax. Has that been resolved and when can I expect to receive notice that my account is now clear?"

Compare this to the following:

"Yeah, I just got another big bill from you guys. I called there about a month or two ago and talked to a lady that said my doctor's office screwed up and that you guys weren't going to pay unless they fixed it and I called my doctor's office and they said it's your fault and I am not going to pay $4800 because you guys screwed up. So are you going to take care of this or should I sue you?"

Take Charge

Use people's names. Thank them by name and take the time to remember their names. It makes a huge difference in getting someone to go the extra mile to solve your problem. It also informs them that you are paying attention and know whom to blame if something goes wrong or if they give you incorrect information.

The types of details that you will want to write down include the time and date of the conversation, and the name and title of the persons you spoke with and what they said (what they told you to do, what the problem was, what they promised to do). In addition, you should write down what you said to them, especially what you said you would do. You should also make sure to take notes of specific follow-up items—who should you contact, as well as when and how (by letter, fax, e-mail, or phone) you should contact this person, or if someone will be contacting you (who, when, and how).

Principle 6: Put it all together and go after what you want.

In most cases, you can get what you want if you go about it the right way. In other cases, you can at least get to better. Applying these ideals and techniques to any interaction of consequence will ensure that you have laid the groundwork for the best possible solution. You will not have to clean up any messes to keep moving forward. Everything will be clean, logical, calm, and dignified. You will allow people to help you and let them feel good about doing it.

Know Your Rights as a Person With Diabetes

Until diagnosed with diabetes, many people may perceive disability rights as those protections offered to people using mobility devices, are blind or hearing impaired, or coping with other visible "challenges." However, the Americans with Disability Act (ADA) defines physical impairment as:

> Any physiological disorder or condition, cosmetic disfigurement, or anatomical loss affecting one or more of the following body systems: neurological, musculoskeletal, special sense organs, respiratory (including speech organs), cardiovascular, reproductive, digestive, genitourinary, hemic and lymphatic, skin, and endocrine.[1]

One thing that has been controversial and problematic with the original ADA is the definition of "disabled." The original law was intentionally written in broad language around who was protected, mostly focusing on the idea that discrimination for pretty much *any* reason was wrong. Over the years, the definition of "disabled" has become narrower and has excluded many people with manageable conditions, meaning that symptoms could be controlled, such as diabetes, epilepsy, and cancer. In September 2008, President Bush signed the ADA Amendments Act (formerly known as the ADA Restoration Act), which became effective January 1, 2009. This amendment basically reinstates the intended protections, as it says that to be considered a "disability" it doesn't matter if the condition or symptom can be made better or controlled by medication, it doesn't matter if it comes and goes, and it doesn't have to severely restrict major life activities.

Keep in mind that the ADA protects people while they are having problems that limit their ability to function, as well as people who have an illness or disorder that does *not* limit their abilities, but others use as a reason to discriminate. Take a couple minutes to look through the

Web site at *www.ada.gov* to get an idea about what the ADA has meant to people in the United States, and especially to people with diabetes. Go to "Search" in the top menu bar and enter "diabetes" to see the various ways that the ADA has provided protection for people with diabetes to do what they need to do to manage their diabetes while fully participating in society, including attending private school or becoming a police officer.

Check Out "The Patient's Bill of Rights"

I guess my favorite document summing up the "rights" that people in the medical system have is the "Consumer Bill of Rights and Responsibilities" that was adopted by the US Advisory Commission on Consumer Protection and Quality in the Health Care Industry in 1998. It is also known as the "Patient's Bill of Rights." Although these are called "rights," the document itself does not have any binding legal ways to enforce any of them, but instead states: "The rights enumerated in this report can be achieved in several ways including voluntary actions by health plans, purchasers, facilities, and providers; the effects of market forces; accreditation processes; as well as State or Federal legislation or regulation."[2]

Although not legally binding, The Patient's Bill of Rights was created with the right intentions. It was an attempt to give people confidence in the health care system and emphasize the importance of a good relationship between patient and doctor. It also, interestingly enough, laid out patients' responsibilities to ensure that they were acting as responsible participants in getting the most from their medical care.

The rights contained in the "Patient's Bill of Rights" are summarized as follows:

Information disclosure. You have the right to receive all necessary information about your health plan, doctors, and facilities in a format that you can understand so that you can make informed decisions about your health care.

Choice of providers and plans. You have the right to choose the insurance plan and the doctors that are right for your situation.

Access to emergency services. If your health is in immediate danger, you have the right to be stabilized using emergency services without needing to wait for authorization or incurring extra costs.

Participation in treatment decisions. You have the right to know and understand your options for treatment and participate in decisions about your care, as well as be represented by loved ones if you are unable to make these decisions yourself.

Respect and nondiscrimination. You have the right to receive respectful, nondiscriminatory care from your doctors and insurance representatives.

Confidentiality of health information. You have the right to have your health care information kept confidential and protected. You also have the right to read and have a copy your own medical record. You have the right to request that incorrect, irrelevant, or incomplete information be changed in your file.

Complaints and appeals. You have the right to a quick and objective review of any complaint you have against your insurance company, doctors and other medical personnel, or facilities. This includes complaints about waiting times and operating hours, how you are treated by medical staff, the adequacy of clinics and hospitals, and other complaints.

Responsibilities as a Person With Diabetes

An interesting part of the Patients' Bill of Rights is the "Statement of Responsibilities":

> In a health care system that protects consumers' rights, it is reasonable to expect and encourage consumers to assume reasonable responsibilities. Greater individual involvement by consumers in their care increases the likelihood of achieving the best outcomes and helps support a quality improvement, cost-conscious environment.[2]

Such responsibilities include making an effort to

- Take responsibility for maximizing healthy habits, such as exercising, not smoking, and eating a healthy diet;
- Become involved in specific health care decisions;
- Work collaboratively with health care providers in developing and carrying out agreed-upon treatment plans;

- Disclose relevant information and clearly communicate wants and needs;
- Use the health plan's internal complaint and appeal processes to address concerns that may arise;
- Avoid knowingly spreading disease;
- Recognize the reality of risks and limits of the science of medical care and the human fallibility of the health care professional;
- Be aware of a health care provider's obligation to be reasonably efficient and equitable in providing care to other patients and the community;
- Become knowledgeable about his or her health plan coverage and health plan options (when available) including all covered benefits, limitations, and exclusions, rules regarding use of network providers, coverage and referral rules, appropriate processes to secure additional information, and the process to appeal coverage decisions;
- Show respect for other patients and health workers;
- Make a good faith effort to meet financial obligations;
- Abide by administrative and operational procedures of health plans, health care providers, and government health benefit programs; and
- Report wrongdoing and fraud to appropriate resources or legal authorities.

I find this part of the Patient's Bill of Rights interesting—it's almost like a mix between a guide to patient etiquette and a prenuptial agreement between the patient and the health care system. Although I see obvious areas of "CYA" (cover your ass) to provide ethical loopholes for medical professionals and the industry as a whole if abused, many of the points are worth remembering and pursuing in our interactions with the health care system.

Understand the Politics of Diabetes

When considering government politics and policies that impact our lives, and that we might be able to influence them in some way, it is important to realize that decisions get made on three levels—federal, state, and city or local levels. It is not always immediately clear who is deciding what and what the decision actually means, as states often have loopholes and budgets to allow them to do "their own thing" in many situations. Cities and towns also vary in their implementation of state policy, and even in adhering to their own regulations, citing budgetary reasons, or claiming that an improvement is in the pipeline. Hell, even landlords and owners of individual establishments can avoid complying to code if no one is paying attention. The message here is that you have to dig around to find out what is going on, what the law says and what advocates want to change, who is the "target" for getting the change made, and how to best reach that person.

To find out what is really cooking in terms of active federal legislation around diabetes, go to *www.GovTrack.us* and enter "diabetes" (in quotation marks) in the "Bill Search" field. The information there is just as it is described on the Web site:

> GovTrack.us is an independent tool to help the public research and track the activities in the U.S. Congress, promoting government transparency and civic education through novel uses of technology. You'll find here the status of U.S. federal legislation, voting records in the Senate and House of Representatives, and information on Members of Congress, as well as congressional committees and the Congressional Record.[3]

The site also has the full text of all the bills listed. The very best thing about this Web site, at least for me, is that it really explains each step in the process, as well as the terms used. You can truly figure out what is going on and seem really smart after a visit to GovTrack.us. Much of the same information can be found at THOMAS (*http://thomas.loc.gov*), a service of the Library of Congress.

Issues on a State or Local Level

Federal policies are important and often determine what happens in our individual lives, but often we are immediately impacted by things regulated on a state level or by our municipal (city or town) governing bodies. Politics around things like affordable housing, accessible transportation, vouchers for respite care, and reducing premiums for state high-risk pool insurance may be "hot tickets" at different times in your state or city. In addition, many issues will be represented by organizations that hold meetings or send out newsletters around the topic and can tell you how you can get involved.

> ### Take Charge
>
> You must understand who has the authority to make a change. Try not to waste your efforts anywhere else.

Because we are all individuals with our own unique needs and values, there is no way to provide a comprehensive overview of the issues impacting the lives of everyone with diabetes. However, there are a handful of topics that are pretty specific to diabetes or could have a considerable impact on the lives of many of us living with the disease. I have pulled together a little "primer" to help you understand or to remind you of some of the things that diabetes advocates are calling for at the time of this writing.

> ### Gratitude Moment
>
> An advocate is a person who supports and works toward achieving a specific goal. Lucky for us, there are lots of diabetes advocates out there. Consider joining them in their fights—they already know the right people and have developed strategies. Add your voice to theirs.

> ### Make It Better
>
> In some cases, it takes as few as 5 or 10 letters from real people to influence a senator or get his or her attention. Don't underestimate yourself or your potential impact.

Issue: Restricted Access to Private Insurance and Other Issues Around Affordable Health Care

What Is the Issue and What Do Advocates Want?

Until the signing of the Patient Protection and Affordable Care Act and the Health Care and Education Affordability Act of 2010 (a.k.a. the "health care reform law") that was signed in March 2010, those of us with diabetes could be denied health coverage by insurance carriers, which use "preexisting conditions" as a way of turning people down who apply for policies. This had several ramifications. Some of us stay in jobs that we dislike or that are too physically demanding for fear that we will be unable to get or afford health insurance coverage if we leave them. Those of us who have to leave jobs, are self-employed or were never covered end up in the position of not having health insurance at all or paying far higher premiums to our state's "high-risk pool" insurance, which currently carries high deductibles and premiums costing double the regular private insurance (although this is supposed to be addressed under the new law, as well). Needless to say, there are many implications for this, as people end up unable to afford health care or limit utilization to save money.

Advocates wanting "guaranteed eligibility," whereby health insurance companies would have to approve anyone, regardless of health condition, got their wish. However, this provision does not go into effect until 2014. There is plenty of time for further debate and the details still need to be worked out, meaning that there are countless advocacy opportunities as these laws move from "broad ideals" to "real life."

How Do I Find Out More or Get Involved?

These are just a few of the proposed ideas to work toward accessible health care—each of the ideas has its own advocacy groups and supporters. A good place to start learning about these issues is Families USA (*www.familiesusa.org*), an organization that touts itself as "The Voice for Health Care Consumers." The Web site contains tons of information about the different issues with a special section called "Health Reform Central: The Road to Implementation" that gives details as to progress on meeting provisions in the law, as well as a link to "Roadblocks," which attempts to repeal or nullify the new law. The site also links to individual state pages listing advocacy organizations in each state and news about the various health coverage issues in each state.

Also, the American Diabetes Association has an excellent Web site at http://main.diabetes.org/site/PageServer?pagename=diabetes_health _care_reform_now (or just enter "diabetes health care reform" into your search engine) covering exactly what health care reform means for people with diabetes.

Know Your Stuff

To be an effective advocate, you need to learn about both sides of an issue. Be able to debate also. This will enable you to explain your views much better and be much more convincing.

Issue: An Artificial Pancreas Is Within Reach, but Not Available Right Now

What Is the Issue and What Do Advocates Want?

Put simply, people want a cure for diabetes. At this moment in time, there isn't one—however, there are technologies that are close to making life much easier for people with diabetes, especially type 1 diabetes. An "artificial pancreas" is a combination of an insulin pump and a continuous glucose monitor that have been integrated to work together to mimic the insulin delivery of a pancreas in response to fluctuations in blood glucose. Although some people may not consider this a "cure" in the strictest sense of the word, an artificial pancreas would be an exciting development, as it could come pretty close to delivering appropriate amounts of insulin without guesswork or human error.

Of course, although the components are available (insulin pumps and continuous glucose monitoring system [CGMS]), there will have to be adaptations and clinical trials to get them working together "just right," while minimizing the risk of malfunction. There will also have to be quite a bit of effort to get insurance companies to pay for them and to educate clinicians and patients themselves on using this technology.

How Do I Find Out More or Get Involved?

The Juvenile Diabetes Research Foundation International (JDRF) is really leading the advocacy effort around the artificial pancreas and stem cell approaches. The goal of the Artificial Pancreas Project of JDRF is "an artificial pancreas that will enable a person with diabetes to maintain normal glucose levels by providing the right amount of insulin at the right time, just as the pancreas does in individuals without diabetes."[4] To do this, they are working to fund research around the world and educate stakeholders (government officials, insurance executives, and doctors) about these technologies. You can learn more about developments and get involved by visiting *www.artificialpancreasproject.com.*

Issue: Home Blood Glucose Monitors Not Accurate

What Is the Issue and What Do Advocates Want?

Studies published in the last couple of years have shown that blood glucose monitors can deliver results that vary from results obtained in the laboratory by more than the Food and Drug Administration (FDA) standard of within 20%, which many experts still think is unacceptable.[5] Even the +/− 20% deviation can lead to more instances of hypoglycemia and high blood glucose, as people rely on these faulty numbers to make decisions to prevent these occurrences. People in industry (the manufacturers of the blood glucose meters) claim that they could probably live with standards that tightened accuracy to within 15% of true laboratory values, but that anything more accurate than that is not possible using current technology (or at least would not allow them to produce a meter that would be priced competitively).

How Do I Find Out More or Get Involved?

Although this issue seems pretty straightforward, there are many different steps to getting these standards changed, much less translated into more accurate meters for the masses. There are many people out in the online world who are keeping up with this issue and working to get comments in the FDA from people with diabetes—the very people who rely on accurate numbers to make decisions about insulin doses and actions they are going to take to maintain tight blood glucose control. A couple of notes are from Kelly Kunik (*http://diabetesaliciousness.blogspot.com*) and Kerri Morrone Sparling (*www.sixuntilme.com*). You can also try entering "inaccurate blood glucose meters" into your search engine. You will have to sift through some stuff, but eventually it will happen on a blog entry that will get you caught up with what is happening and give you ideas on how to help, whom to complain to, or what to demand.

Issue: Access to Diabetes Prevention and Care Is Not Equal

What Is the Issue, and What Do Advocates Want?

Some minority ethnic groups, including Hispanic/Latinos, African Americans, Asian Americans, Native Hawaiian and other Pacific Islanders, and American Indians and Alaskan Natives are impacted harder by diabetes. These groups not only have a higher incidence of diabetes, but they also are much more likely to have serious complications from diabetes. There are many factors contributing to this disparity, including access to medical care, lower health literacy, and socioeconomic issues are some of the main contributors. Cultural norms and attitudes toward health (including diabetes) also interact with these factors. These problems lead to poor adherence to medication and other treatment regimens, unhealthy food choices, and infrequent visits to the doctor. Advocates want this to change—that work is to be done to educate people about diabetes within their community. And that work takes money.

How Do I Find Out More or Get Involved?

The H.R. 1995, otherwise known as the Eliminating Disparities in Diabetes Prevention Access and Care Act, is designed to address this health inequality by "promoting research, treatment, and education regarding diabetes in minority populations."[6] You can get involved by writing to your members of Congress and asking them to support this bill. The American Diabetes Association makes it pretty easy for you by providing an electronic form to fill out and send. You can find information about this bill and the progress that is being made by going to the American Diabetes Association's Web site (*www.diabetes.org*) and entering "disparities" in the search field at the upper right corner of the page.

Be an Activist

For all of the undesirable health stuff that is part of the diabetes package, we are truly fortunate to have strong organizations behind us. When it comes to advocacy, the JDRF is at the forefront for people with type 1 diabetes, with formal activist and volunteer programs set up across the country. Visit their site at *www.jdrf.org* to learn about advocacy opportunities, and approaches. The American Diabetes Association has a place on their Web site (*www.diabetes.org*) where people can learn to "advocate for change" around diabetes issues, which is more inclusive of people with type 2 diabetes.

Participating in programs set up by existing organizations gives us the opportunity to either jump right in to full-fledged lobbying or try out volunteering by assisting with education campaigns or fundraising events. There are other organizations, both those that are diabetes-specific, as well as those focused on other issues, that would also welcome our voices and participation with open arms.

Take Charge

Be an activist. Direct your frustration into effectively making things better.

Make It Better

Although many people think of activists as those people who are screaming, protesting, and resisting arrest to get a point across, I have a broader definition. I think an activist is anyone who puts effort toward making things better in the world. Activists are those people who lick envelopes, who hold strangers' hands, and who deliver meals.

Whether you are more of a "screamer" or an "envelope licker," get involved. We need all the help we can get.

Other Opportunities to Take Action

Maybe you want to do something, but aren't sure that hanging out with politicians or lobbying on "the hill" is for you. Some of the opportunities that came up when I did a search are less about lobbying and more about helping people in a more direct way or helping organizations with logistics at their events. They included the following:

Diabetes camp volunteer. The American Diabetes Association runs a large number of summer camps for kids with diabetes. There are plenty of volunteer opportunities at the individual camps, from being a counselor to helping with different activities to working in the office. This is a great way to inspire and be inspired by these children. For more information, click on the "Living With Diabetes" tab at *www.diabetes.com* and look on the menu for "ADA Camps."

Volunteer for the Stop Diabetes! movement of the American Diabetes Association. To find out about opportunities in your area, call 1-800-DIABETES (800-342-2383). There might be chances to help with logistics at a diabetes expo or at one of the fund-raising events in your city.

Volunteer mentors. Some chapters and branches of the JDRF run mentor programs to pair families of children who have been living with type 1 diabetes with people whose child is newly diagnosed with type 1 diabetes to offer emotional support and answers to nonmedical questions. Contact your local office of JDRF or call the main office at 800-533-CURE (800-533-2873) for more information.

LINCS (Linking Individuals in Need With Care and Services) volunteer counselors. This is a program of the Medicare Rights Center that trains volunteers to help people navigate the Medicare system, including determining eligibility and filling out forms and applications. Volunteers provide this help by phone from their own homes. To find out more about this program, visit the Web site at *www.medicarerights.org* or contact the LINCS program coordinators at 212-204-6273 or e-mail LINCS@medicarerights.org.

Fund-raising Opportunities

One easy way to "get your feet wet" in getting involved with organizations helping people is to help raise money for these organizations to continue their work. It is a good way to meet people and make friends with an interest in diabetes, or another issue close to your heart, as well as to scope out the organization and get a feel for it before getting more involved. Here are a couple of ways that you can offer support:

Participate in an event or support an event. These days, it seems like people don't really just write checks anymore. Instead, they ride their bicycles 150 miles, walk or run various distances, golf, dance, or do all sorts of other things to raise money. If you are physically up to the challenge, participating in one of these events can be really fun and a great way to remind yourself of the effort that people are putting in to support diabetes research and programs (although many people participate for the sheer physical challenge and have little interest in the benefitting organization). If you are not overly excited about the idea of riding a bicycle uphill for 2 days, there are usually plenty of opportunities to volunteer to support the event participants or assist with logistics, both leading up to and on event day. Your help will be hugely appreciated if you are willing to do boring tasks, like stuff envelopes or compile information packets for participants.

Volunteer to help with fund-raising. Some organizations and chapters have well-run volunteer programs and will be thrilled to let you do something to raise money or raise awareness, such as sending out preprinted letters requesting donations or staffing a booth at a big gathering.

Hold your own event to raise money for your favorite organization. This can be a really fun thing to do to help raise funds for an organization— pretty much "the sky's the limit" in terms of thinking about what kind of event to hold. You can have a simple cocktail party for several people, during which you speak about your own experience with diabetes and ask for a donation. Or, you can put together a large picnic and invite people from your church to bring food. You can get together with your friends and hold a bake sale, a bowling tournament, or a garage sale, with the proceeds going to your favorite organization. It is very important to let people you invite to participate, especially in the social events, and know that this is a fund-raiser, and they will be asked for money. This can help avoid any awkwardness around "making the ask."

The Bottom Line

When many people hear the words *advocacy* or *activism*, they picture people screaming and holding placards, fighting for the right to life, the right to choose, the rights of prisoners not to die, the rights of the terminally ill to assisted suicide, and so forth. However, these words—advocacy and activism—can also mean calmly figuring out what is not right in the world for ourselves or others, and quietly and methodically working to fix it. It can take the form of letters written to people in power, a request for a second opinion if you are not satisfied with a doctor's answer, or helping parents of a child with diabetes educate teachers and classmates about this disease to make sure that they can see past it.

Activism for health reasons exploded into the public eye at the height of the AIDS crisis. Everyone was very frightened of this new disease, blame was everywhere, and people simply did not know what to do. People were divided in their views, and in many cases, discrimination deepened. In the 20-plus years since the virus first made an appearance in the United States, think how far we have come.

Two decades later, things are different for all of us with health problems, including those of us living with diabetes. Besides people with diabetes, many other individuals who may have once kept information and fears about their illness to themselves out of embarrassment or fear of being misunderstood have found their voices and come together to speak up and speak out. These include, among others, cancer survivors, people with mental illness, and parents of children with disabilities. They demand equality, inclusion in society, that resources be directed toward research, that the flaws in the health care system be remedied, and that they be allowed to live with dignity.

In his book *Strong at the Broken Places* that profiles five people living with different chronic illnesses, Richard Cohen says calmly, but firmly, "These are the faces of illness in America. Do not look away. The characters may surprise you, even shatter a stereotype or two. They are people, not cases, survivors, not victims."[7]

As people and as survivors, we *can* make a big difference, especially if we work together. We can make a difference for ourselves and for those who cannot speak for themselves. We can be strengthened in our shared experience and make this experience the very best it can be.

Conclusion: The *Bottom* Bottom Line

As I draw closer to ending this book, I have been losing sleep over what you, the reader, will take away from it.

I set out to tell the truth about diabetes—at the very least, I wanted to share *my* truth about living with diabetes. In pouring that truth onto the page, I alternatively worried that my "reality dump" was destroying hope and that my calls to action were giving the impression that I wanted everyone reading my words to become "full-time diabetics."

Neither of these was my intention. Hope is what keeps me going—not uninformed optimism, but hope that is founded in the progress around this disease that I have seen in my lifetime and what I have been able to do for myself. As for making diabetes the star of the show, this is the last thing that I want to see anyone do: We are all far more interesting than our diabetes. Do not let diabetes erode your personality by letting it take over your every thought and action. Manage it and put it in its place.

I will acknowledge, however, that I am fortunate, yet life with diabetes is still extremely hard. I have a loving family, partner, and friends. I have access to the best medical care in this country. I can afford treatment and I have good insurance coverage. I have a good survival instinct and healthy self-confidence around my ability to manage this disease. Yet, many people are missing one or more of these crucial components to living successfully with a chronic illness. They must be fortified and encouraged.

There are many things about diabetes that are beyond my control. However, there are things that are within my influence. For instance, I strive for tight control of my glucose levels. This has not prevented me from temporary blindness or gastroparesis. Contrary to popular myths, some complications just happen to some people, regardless of how vigilant they are about their diet or monitoring their glucose levels. This is not their fault.

When I die, I do not want anyone to say to my loved ones that I didn't take care of myself. I want those who care about me to know that I did my very best, and that I lived life to the fullest without surrendering to this disease. I want them to know that I lived a great life despite my diabetes.

References

Chapter 2

1. Weiss MA, Funnel MM. *Little Book of Diabetes That You Need to Read.* Philadelphia, PA: Running Press; 1997.

2. National Diabetes Information Clearinghouse. Diabetes overview. Available at: http://diabetes.niddk.nih.gov/dm/pubs/overview/. Accessed July 16, 2010.

3. The *Journal of Clinical Investigation* on April 19, 2010, and will appear in the May print edition of the journal.

4. Butler AE, Janson J, Bonner-Weir S, Ritzel R, Rizza RA, Butler PC. Beta-cell deficit and increased beta-cell apoptosis in humans with type 2 diabetes. *Diabetes.* 2003;52(1):102–10.

5. dLife. *Type 2 diabetes.* Available at: http://www.dlife.com/diabetes/information//type-2/diabetes-causes/index.html. Accessed July 16, 2010.

6. McCulloch DK. *The Diabetes Answer Book.* Naperville, IL: Sourcebooks, Inc; 2008.

7. Yeh HC, Duncan BB, Schmidt MI, Wang NY, Brancati FL. Smoking, smoking cessation, and the risk for type 2 diabetes mellitus: a cohort study. *Ann Intern Med.* 2010;152:10–17.

8. Diabetes overview of the national diabetes clearinghouse. Available at: http://diabetes.niddk.nih.gov/dm/pubs/overview/#other. Accessed September 15, 2010.

9. Centers for Disease Control and Prevention. Number of people with diabetes increases to 24 Million. Available at: http://www.cdc.gov/media/pressrel/2008/r080624.htm. Accessed July 16, 2010.

10. American Association of Clinical Endocrinologists. Implementation conference for ACE outpatient diabetes mellitus consensus conference recommendations: position statement. Paper presented February 2, 2005; Washington, DC.

11. Reynolds RM, Strachan MW. Home blood glucose monitoring in type 2 diabetes. *BMJ*. 2004;329(7469):754–755. Available at: http://www.bmj.com /cgi/content/full/329/7469/754. Accessed July 16, 2010.

Chapter 3

1. McCulloch DK. *The Diabetes Answer Book*. Naperville, IL: Sourcebooks, Inc; 2008.

2. Swinnen SG, Hoekstra JB, DeVries JH. Insulin therapy for type 2 diabetes. *Diabetes Care* [serial online]. 2009; 32(Suppl 2): S253–S259. Available at: http://care.diabetesjournals.org/content/32/suppl_2/S253.full. Accessed July 16, 2010.

3. Buckingham B, Wilson DM, Lecher T, Hanas R, Kaiserman K, Cameron F. Duration of nocturnal hypoglycemia prior to seizures. *Diabetes Care* [serial online]. 2008; 31(11): 2110–2112. Available at: http://care.diabetesjournals.org /content/early/2008/08/11/dc08-0863. Accessed July 16, 2010.

4. Kolata G. Diabetes heart treatments may cause harm. [New York Times Web site] March 14, 2010. Available at: http://www.nytimes.com/2010/03/15 /health/research/15heart.html. Accessed July 16, 2010.

5. Kolata G. Diabetes heart treatments may cause harm. [New York Times Web site] March 14, 2010. Available at: http://www.nytimes.com/2010/03/15/health /research/15heart.html. Accessed July 16, 2010.

6. American Diabetes Association. Standards of medical care in diabetes— 2010. *Diabetes Care*. 2010;33(suppl 1): S11–S61.

7. Buse J. Statin treatment in diabetes mellitus. *Clin Diabetes*. [serial online]. 2003; 21(4): 168–172. Available at: http://clinical.diabetesjournals.org /content/21/4/168.long. Accessed July 16, 2010.

8. Number of U.S. transplants per year, 1988–2008. Infoplease website. Available at: http://www.infoplease.com/science/health/us-transplants-year-1988-2007 .html. Accessed July 16, 2010.

9. Anderson RJ, Lustman PJ, Clouse RE, et al. Prevalence of depression in adults with diabetes: a systematic review. *Diabetes*. 2000; 49(Suppl 1): A64.

Chapter 4

1. Diabetes education. American Association of Diabetes Educators website. Available at: http://www.diabeteseducator.org/DiabetesEducation/Definitions .html. Accessed July 16, 2010.

Chapter 5

1. Karter AJ, Subramanian U, Saha C, et al. Barriers to insulin initiation: The translating research into action for diabetes insulin starts project. *Diabetes Care*. 2010;33(4):733–735.

2. Diabetes drug prescribed when contraindicated–metformin. *Nutr Health Rev* [serial online]. Available at: http://findarticles.com/p/articles/mi_m0876 /is_85/ai_106027145/. Accessed July 16, 2010.

3. Barron J, Wahl P, Fisher M, Plauschinat C. Effect of prescription copayments on adherence and treatment failure with oral antidiabetic medications. *PT*. 2008;33(9):532–553.

4. Hunt J, Rozenfeld Y, Shenolikar R. Effect of patient medication cost share on adherence and glycemic control. *Manag Care*. 2009;18(7):47–53.

5. Brunton S. Beyond glycemic control: treating the entire type 2 diabetes disorder. *Postgrad Med*. 2009;121(5):68–81.

6. Peyrot M, Skovlund SE, Landgraf R. Epidemiology and correlates of weight worry in the multinational Diabetes Attitudes, Wishes and Needs study. *Curr Med Res Opin*. 2009;25(8):1985–1993.

7. Hauber AB, Mohamed AF, Johnson FR, Falvey H. Treatment preferences and medication adherence of people with Type 2 diabetes using oral glucose-lowering agents. *Diabet Med*. 2009;26(4):416-424.

8. Dirmaier J, Watzke B, Koch U, et al. Diabetes in primary care: prospective associations between depression, nonadherence and glycemic control. *Psychother Psychosom*. 2010;79(3):172–8.

9. Egede LE, Ellis C. Development and psychometric properties of the 12-item diabetes fatalism scale. *J Gen Intern Med*. 2010;25(1):61–6.

Chapter 6

1. Knutson KL, Ryden AM, Mander BA, Van Cauter E. Role of sleep duration and quality in the risk and severity of type 2 diabetes mellitus. *Arch Intern Med*. 2006;166(16):1768–74.

2. Knutson KL. Impact of sleep and sleep loss on glucose homeostasis and appetite regulation. *Sleep Med Clin*. 2007; 2(2): 187–197.

Chapter 7

1. Bunker K. Tips on finding a job when you have diabetes. *Diabetes Forecast*. December 2009. Available at: http://forecast.diabetes.org/magazine /your-ada/tips-finding-job-when-you-have-diabetes. Accessed August 07, 2010.

Chapter 10

1. Americans with Disabilities Act of 1990, Pub L No. 101-336, §2, 104 Stat 328 (1991).

2. President's Advisory Commission on Consumer Protection and Quality in the Health Care Industry. *Consumer Bill of Rights and Responsibilities*. Washington, DC: The Commission; 1997.

3. GovTrack.us Web site. Available at: http://www.govtrack.us/about.xpd. Accessed September 15, 2010.

4. Artificial Pancreas Project. JDRF website. Available at: http:// advocacy.jdrf.org/index.cfm?page_id=109568. Accessed September 15, 2010.

5. Kimberly MM, Vesper HW, Caudill SP, et al. Variability among five over-the-counter blood glucose monitors. *Clin Chim Acta*. 2006;364(1–2):292–297.

6. Eliminating Disparities in Diabetes Prevention Access and Care Act, H.R. 1995, 111th Cong. (2009).

7. Cohen RM. *Strong at the Broken Places: Voices of Illness, a Chorus of Hope*. New York, NY: HarperCollins Publisher; 2008.

Index

Note: Throughout the Index, the abbreviation ABMS is used for American Board of Medical Specialties; ADA for American Diabetes Association; CAM for complementary and alternative medicine; CDE for certified diabetes educator; CGMS for continuous glucose monitoring system; DRP for Diabetes Recognition Program; GFR for glomerular filtration rate; HDL for high-density lipoprotein; HHNS for hyperosmolar hyperglycemic nonketotic syndrome; ICA/GADA for islet cell antibodies/glutamic acid decarboxylase 65 antibodies; JDRF for Juvenile Diabetes Research Foundation; LADA for latent autoimmune diabetes in adults; LGBT for lesbian, gay, bisexual transgender; NPH for neutral protamine Hagedorn; PAD for peripheral artery disease and PDR for *Physician's Desk Reference*. Page number followed by *n* indicates footnote.